RADICALLY FREE

THE ANTI-INFLAMMATORY AND ANTIOXIDANT SOLUTION TO WEIGHT MANAGEMENT AND WELLNESS

By

MACHIEL N. KENNEDY, M.D,

Diplomate ABFM and ABOM

STEVEN E. WARREN, M.D., DPA

CIME, FABFP, FABHPM, FAPWCA,

Diplomate ABFM

ENDORSEMENTS

I feel that *Radically Free* represents a very significant book, as it combines practical medical advice based on very solid biochemical foundation to address the growing epidemic of obesity and its associated diseases. It is not lack of willpower, but lack of our management of excess free radicals and inflammation that is driving our obesity crisis. I consider this to be a must-read book for everyone.

Dr. Barry Sears
Author of The Zone

Radically Free answers all your questions about how and why healthy eating is important. The idea of obesity being an inflammatory disease makes sense, and this book brings the solution to a clear, workable solution. The humor and matter-of-fact presentation cover a lot of information in a concise and readable manner. If someone you care about is struggling to justify a change in their food choices, hand them a copy of *Radically Free* and then wait for their "aha" moment.

Vicki Berkus MD, PhD, CEDS

Radically Free is a fascinating account of the science of inflammation and antioxidants and their contribution to weight management and wellness. *Radically Free* is an invaluable contribution to the national conversation about the obesity epidemic. Prepare to be educated!

Ralph E. Carson, PhD, RD

Radically Free is much more than a play on words. The content of the book is a brilliant insight into the science and psychology of our ability to transform our physical and emotional condition. *Radically Free* is not a book for the person who wants a magical pill or empty words and "Photoshopped" pictures of people the author or publisher wants you to believe you could look like if you buy this book or that product. If you want to be "radically free," this book is for you. Radical desire to understand mentally plus radical desire to change physical behavior will result in a *Radically Free* life!

Dr. Terry L. Collier
Executive director of the Anona Family Life Counseling Center

TABLE OF CONTENTS

FOREWORD

How would you love to dive into a pool of chocolate and come out thin? It definitely sounds fun, but unrealistic, you say. How can you dive into a chocolate pool and change your appearance and how you feel? Scientists and doctors have listed chocolate as an evil food that causes a multitude of medical problems. Chocolate will make you fat, increase your acne, cause kidney stones, or hurt your stomach, etc. No one could believe that eating chocolate would make you thin. This must be a joke. Can chocolate and weight loss go in the same sentence? That is definitely a paradox.

The truth is that the cocoa bean, along with many other anti-inflammatory and antioxidant foods, has the ability to make you lose weight, improve your mood, stabilize your health, and maximize your quality of life. *How?*

In this book we are going to explore the problem of obesity and how we got there. We are going to discuss the nutrients you need to help you function more effectively and efficiently. We want you to have a perfectly tuned body. We will discuss how we are sabotaging our metabolism. We will help you understand the simple formula of calories in and calories out in planning your health maintenance. We all have been on thousands of diets, but have we made any headway? If it were simple to reduce calories by not eating as much and increase calories through exercise, we would all be thin. Guess what? It's not happening! Why?

We want to explore the health benefits of an anti-inflammatory, high-antioxidant health-maintenance plan. We will discuss how a diet teeming with antioxidants will boost your health and as a side effect help you lose fat. Losing weight is a side effect? *Wow!*

Your skin will improve, your mood will improve, your heart will improve, and as a matter of fact, most everything in your body will improve on an anti-inflammatory and high-antioxidant plan.

We will help you understand how you can incorporate this simple plan into your daily regimen and be successful for the first time in your life. It is a plan that you can do without any feeling of let-down, depression, weakness, or guilt.

We will show you how to stop that carbohydrate (carb) craving, decrease the perception of achiness in your body, and eat the right proportions. This is not a fad diet, a single nutrient diet, or a starvation diet. It is a simple way of eating properly with the addition of an anti-inflammatory and high-antioxidant meal system that will make you the best you can be.

So, join the "A" Team and become radically free.

Steve Warren, MD
2010

INTRODUCTION

My Story - Dr. Kennedy

I was a fat kid.

Actually, you could say that by the time I was in fourth grade, I had become obese. My parents had moved us from the house where I grew up, and to compensate for lack of friends and a new environment, I ate. Food became my friend and companion. It wouldn't leave; it stuck around. Boy, did it stick to all the wrong places.

I can remember coming home after school and getting ready to watch my favorite TV shows. Of course, this meant getting a huge bowl of ice cream with a caramel topping and whipped cream (hold the cherry, I am watching my weight). It was great to settle into an afternoon of TV and treats. Exercise and activity were almost nonexistent.

My posture and my gait got progressively worse, because I led with my stomach, so I ended up waddling around with my feet doing a duck walk. I created my own world and lived there where nothing was wrong.

This attitude lasted through junior high and into high school, when I finally decided that I wanted more out of life. Namely, I wanted to date girls, and the way I looked and felt would not cut it. Of course, I was slow to stop overeating and start dieting, because the pleasures of food always seemed to win out. In addition, a great ability to rationalize my environment helped.

By the end of high school I had corrected the weight problem and was doing better. By the time I got into college, I was actually at a respectable weight. Of course, the ability to overeat persisted. In fact, to this day it persists and is a demon I constantly battle. I struggled with weight into my adult years. I loved to overindulge in food and could always rationalize that it was OK. When you come from obesity, you learn how rationalization makes everything all right. It was a great deception that kept me from facing the truth.

Early in my medical practice, I discovered something called the Cambridge Diet. It was about 330 calories per day. It was hard to believe that people could survive on so few calories and that it was healthy, so I began researching it and eventually decided to use it in my office. The response from the patients was good, but I still did not feel comfortable using it. I began looking for an alternative program and found it. It was called the Optifast Diet. After using it in my office for a year with moderately good success, I decided to take it into the hospital. The hospital was reluctant at first to take on such a drastic diet plan, but since there was such good science backing it, they changed their minds. Thus began my weight-loss practice and a lifelong interest in helping others lose weight.

Of course, I can guess what you are thinking; the "fat kid" goes on to become a "fat-doctor."

The hospital made me medical director, and we opened the weight-loss clinic. We were getting about one call a week in the late fall, when Oprah announced that she had lost sixty-five pounds on the Optifast program. That is all it took. We started receiving literally over two hundred calls per day from people demanding to be on that diet. We accommodated them, and my career in obesity management went into high gear.

In 1999 I discovered a medical society dedicated to obesity and its treatment. It was called the American Society of Bariatric Physicians (ASBP). I joined and one year later sat for my boards in bariatrics. I became a board-certified bariatrician and went on to serve on the board for four years, certifying other physicians.

Over the years I have had the pleasure of helping several companies develop weight-loss programs. That became my passion. My goal was to help the world conquer this epidemic known as obesity. I even coined a term—*population-based weight loss*—to help describe my goal.

To me, living at a healthy weight and being healthy are paramount. I wanted to share this dream with others and help them achieve their goals. Obesity is a disease, and a nasty one at that. If we don't conquer it, it will take us down as a nation. It is no laughing matter.

Being someone who has fought obesity all his life, and also has a passion to conquer it, makes me a man on a mission. My mission is to see everyone as a "lean, mean, fat-burning machine."

I also have selfish reasons for doing this. I have lost three of my best friends to obesity-related diseases. These beautiful people left us way too soon because they struggled with this killer disease. I don't want others to have to endure such a terrible loss either. These were my dearest friends, and I miss them.

To this day I struggle with my weight, but I am winning. Weight-related issues will not cause problems with my health. I can do it, and so can you. Just remember that weight loss is not magic; it is hard work and dedication. I challenge you to make the commitment and just do it. I love this quote from a weight-loss participant: "There is so much more to life than being obese."

As the old statement goes, "It is hard by the yard, but a cinch by the inch." Inch your way along to success, and become a winner in the "losing" game.

Remember, it's not about losing. It's about winning. It is about winning the battle with your body. Take our challenge and *win*.

My Story - Dr. Warren

I have always wondered, *How can skinny doctors lecture about obesity and how to lose weight if they never faced the problem themselves?* Obesity in many cases is due to an addiction to food as a stress reducer. As I approached college and dealt with the stresses of academic work, I slowly became a stress eater. I had unlimited access to food in the dorm where I lived. Since I paid for the food, I figured I'd better eat as much as I could. At night after work, my roommate, who worked at a fast-food restaurant, brought home tons of food. Thus I studied, ate, studied, ate, slept for about four hours, and started the pattern over again.

Soon the weight started accumulating. I didn't notice it, as I was stressed trying to get good grades and get into medical school. I lost my perspective of what was important, and I did not take care of myself. I got into medical school after starting a PhD program where I continued my stress eating. I gained a lot of weight and didn't even think about it because I was worried about my grades and learning. I was definitely deceiving myself. The last two years of medical school were a blur: we never slept and ate when we could. We enjoyed all the food we wanted at the cafeteria, and at night we raided the refrigerators on the medical and surgical floors. Because of being up all night and stressed, I ate. Unfortunately, I did not lose my appetite. I ballooned to over three hundred pounds by the time I finished medical school, and I could not figure out why I was so tired.

I went into my residency training weighing a lot. Again I was thrust into a stressful situation and continued to eat and eat. It was a miracle I did not have a heart attack myself whenever a "Code Blue" was called on a patient who was having a heart attack. Because I was on call, I would rush to the bedside to start CPR and coordinate the resuscitation. I was always short of breath, sweating, and exhausted before I even got to the room. I needed the "Code Blue" myself!

At the end of the first year, I was sitting in a medical staff meeting when they introduced the new interns for the next year. Behind me were two older doctors who commented on the new interns. They wondered why the residency program always got fat residents. I was horrified, to say the least. I knew I was one of those "fat" residents and had to do something immediately.

I started a low-carbohydrate diet with a vigorous exercise program. I ate the right types of food and kept track of what I ate. I developed a support system and had the help of many of the staff personnel. Over the next year, I lost over 110 pounds and started doing triathlons, half marathons, and biking long distances. I rode my bike sixty to seventy miles a day. I probably went overboard, but I needed to change my habits regarding stress and food.

Since that time I have fluctuated with my weight but have never let it get out of control without doing something about it. I realize that maintaining your weight is a daily job and is not easy.

When I teach about weight loss and how hard it is to do, I am not that skinny doctor who never had to lose weight, but the doctor who knows.

CHAPTER 1

Medical Conditions Associated with Obesity

Congratulations on Our "Success"

OK! So, we finally did it. The gold medal belongs to the United States. We have become the world's fattest country. Government statistics now tell us that 68 percent of the US population is either overweight or obese. That is a mark that should stand for years.[1]

Not only did we take the world title, but the latest figures from the Center for Disease Control (CDC) also demonstrate that obesity continues to be a significant public-health problem in the US. Just look at this impressive list of health problems associated with weight:

- Coronary heart disease
- Type 2 diabetes
- Cancers (endometrial, breast and colon)

- Hypertension (high blood pressure)
- Dyslipidemia (high total cholesterol or high levels of triglycerides)
- Stroke
- Liver and gallbladder disease
- Sleep apnea and respiratory problems
- Osteoarthritis
- Gynecological problems (abnormal menses, infertility, poly-cystic ovaries)

Folks, we are unstoppable!

But wait! There is more news. As an added bonus, we can also brag about the fact that childhood obesity has more than doubled from 1980 to 2008. An estimated 17 percent of children and adolescents ages two to nineteen years are obese.[2]

Do you remember that one of the health objectives of the national program Healthy People 2010 (HP2010) was to reduce the proportion of adults who are obese to 15 percent? Guess what? We stopped it cold and defeated it. Look at the data. More than one-third of US adults are obese. The prevalence of obesity is 33.8 percent (32.2 percent among men and 35.5 percent among women)![3]

Impressive! Very impressive, but where do we go from here? Judging from the map of obesity, we still have lots of work to do. There are too many states that don't meet the criteria of a body mass index (BMI) of greater than or equal to 30, which is another way of indicating obesity.

Medical Conditions Associated with Obesity

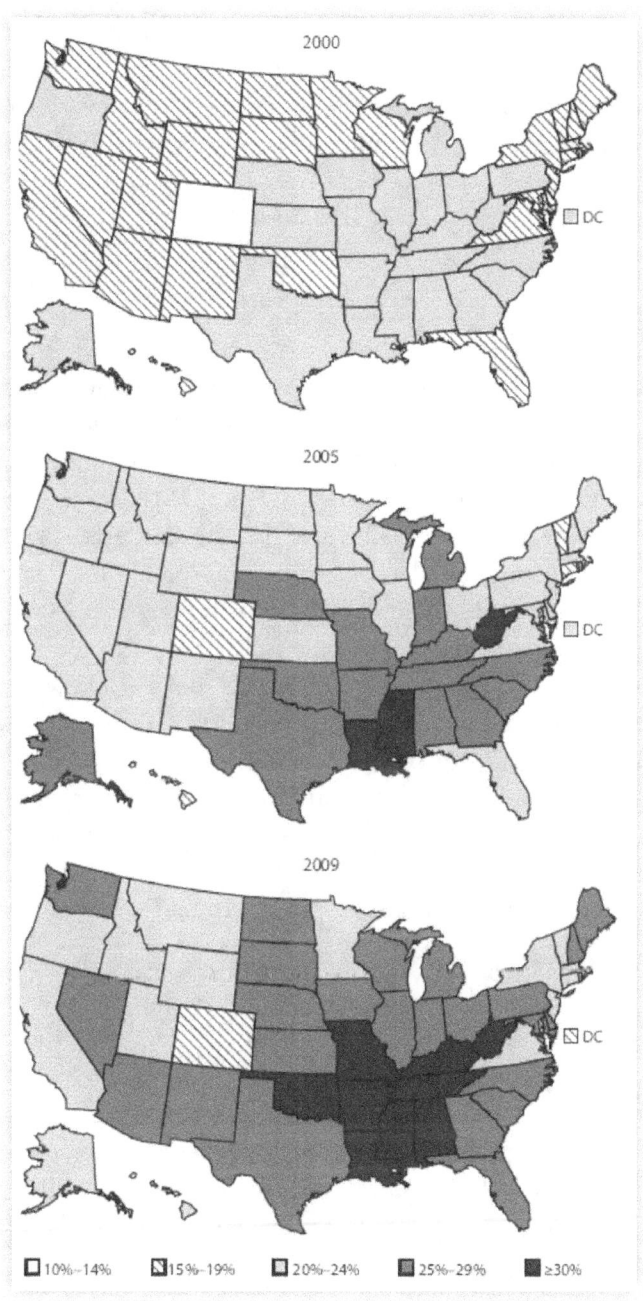

Figure 1-1 shows the growing epidemic of states with ≥30 percent obesity in Black and ≥ 25 percent in dark gray 2000 to 2009.

So, how were we able to gain this world-class reputation? It took lots of work and dedication from many sources and many people, but we did it. Much of our success comes from the fact that Americans are gaining weight on average by 1-3 percent per year. Just think of the legacy we are going to leave our children.

Stop the Presses!

Just released on August 27, 2011, from *The Lancet*, a prestigious British medical journal, we learn more facts. Half of the US population will be obese by 2030 if current trends continue. Currently it is "only" one in three, or 33 percent. Just wait, we can do it. This will cost the US health-care system up to *an extra* $66 billion each year by 2030. The new health-care burden will include an additional million cases of diabetes, 6.8 million additional cases of heart disease and stroke, and over 0.5 million cases of cancer.[4]

These predictions don't have to come true. The article goes on to say that even a modest weight loss at the population level of 1 percent body mass index (BMI) would prevent as many as 2.4 million cases of diabetes and 1.7 million cases of heart disease and stroke.[5]

Let's stop this madness and start on the road to recovery. We can do this through a coordinated effort that includes the private sector (that means you and me).

First we need to understand some basic terminology of how we measure obesity. Here we go.

Body Mass Index (BMI)

Before we can fix the problem of overweight and obesity, we need to understand how these terms are defined. There are two measurements that are easy to understand and calculate with very little equipment. They are body mass index (BMI) and waist circumference.

To determine your BMI, you can use an easy-to-read chart (Appendix A) or you can use this simple formula. Take your weight in pounds and multiply it by 703. Take that number and divide by your height in inches. Take that number and divide by your height in inches again. Confused? Let's do an example.

Suppose someone is five feet four inches (64 inches) tall and weigh 175 pounds.

Multiply 175 pounds by 703   175 pounds X 703 = 123,025

Divide 123,025 by 64 inches   123,025 / 64 inches = 1,922

Divide 1,922 by 64 inches again 1,922 / 64 inches = 30.0 BMI

From our example you learn that this person's BMI is 30.0. Now what does that number mean? The chart below gives the classification of obesity and overweight based on BMI.

Classification	World Health Organization (WHO)	Asia
Underweight	<18.5	
Normal weight	18.5—24.9	18.5—22.9
Overweight	25.0—29.9	23.0—27.4
Obesity class I	30.0—34.9	27.5
Obesity class II	35.0—39.9	
Obesity class III (morbid)	>40.0	

Now looking again at our example, we now know that a BMI of 30 is class I obesity. Be aware that the BMI is accurate for about 85 percent of the population and is an indicator of disease risk and not necessarily aesthetics (it is not about how "hot" you are in a swimsuit but your risk for diseases because of your weight).

The measurement of BMI works for both men and women. Since men carry most of their weight in their belly, which is more dangerous, and women carry most of their weight in their hips and thighs, you can use the same measurement for both sexes. Women can weigh more for the same height because they are at less risk for disease because of their fat distribution.

Remember that obesity puts you at risk for such diseases as strokes, hypertension, diabetes, cancer, heart attacks, and sleep apnea (apart from these diseases, a high BMI is not too serious).

Waist Circumference

Now let's look at the waist circumference. Even if you have an acceptable BMI, an increased waist circumference can put you at the next higher risk for disease. This is true until your BMI reaches 35, and then the combined risks are at their highest.

To measure the waist circumference correctly, stand straight and on the bare skin measure the circumference of your waist just above the wings of the hipbones (iliac crest) on each side of your abdomen. Keep the tape parallel with the floor. It cannot swoop down below your belly. *That is cheating!* This should be about the level of your belly button.

From the chart below, you can see at what measurement the disease risk dramatically increases.

	Caucasian	Asian
Men	$\geq$40 in (102 cm)	$\geq$35 in (88 cm)
Women	$\geq$35 in (90 cm)	$\geq$31 in (80 cm)

Now let's have a reality check, or a "gut check" if you will.

My BMI is _____

My waist circumference is_____

According to these measurements, that makes me _____!

(normal weight, overweight, or obese)

Come on, be honest. You earned the title, so wear it "proudly."

Diseases Associated with Obesity

Most people don't realize that obesity is a disease. It is not a character flaw—it is a major disease. More specifically, it is an inflammatory disease. Think of obesity as a terrorist that has created a "hostile takeover" of your body.

Fat cells of the gut, or belly fat (visceral adiposity), are the most dangerous. That is why the waist circumference measurement is so important. The belly fat cells are not just storage sacks of fat; they are active endocrine glands secreting all kinds of "hostile" chemicals called cytokines into your bloodstream. Most of these cytokines are causing the "hostile takeover." As you can see from Figure 1-3, there are quite a few.

Most of the cytokines cause trouble—except leptin and adiponectin, which are "good guys." Adiponectin is secreted from the fat cells and helps protect the arteries from damage (endothelial protection) and prevents hardening of the arteries (atherosclerosis). As a person gets fatter and fatter, the levels of adiponectin decrease. Conversely, as obesity decreases, your levels of adiponectin increase, and you definitely want them higher.

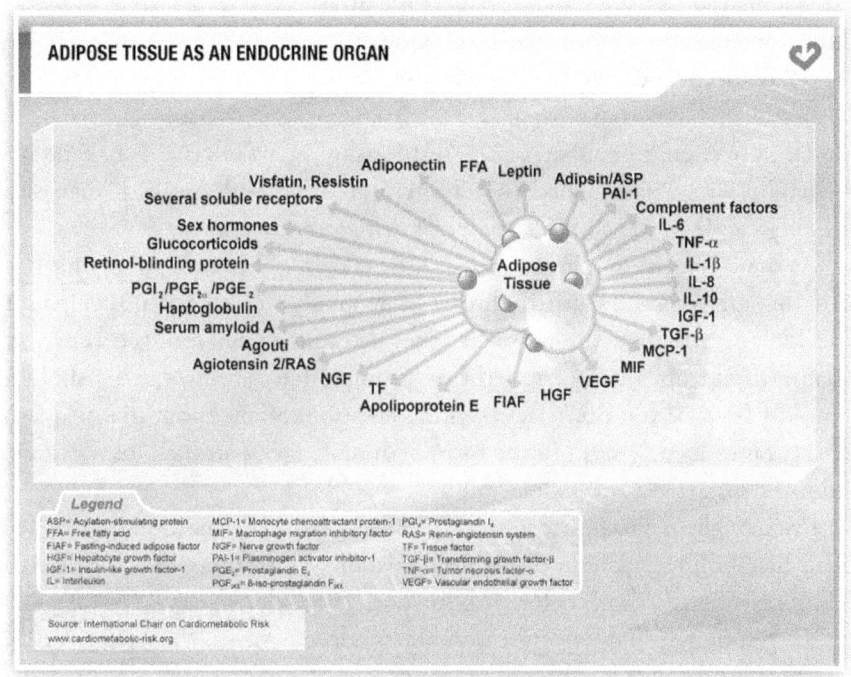

Figure 1-3

It is interesting to note the impressive list of medical complications from obesity. Those cytokines in Figure 1-3 are busy little creatures causing:

Pulmonary Disease
    Hypoventilation Syndrome
    Obstructive Sleep Apnea
Nonalcoholic Fatty Liver Disease
    Steatosis

Intracranial hypertension
Stroke
Cataracts
Coronary Heart Disease
    Type-2 diabetes

Steato-hepatitis	Hypertension
Cirrhosis	Dyslipidemia
Gall Bladder Disease	**Severe Pancreatitis**
Gynecologic Abnormalities	**Cancer**
Irregular periods	Breast, Uterus, Cervix, Colon
Infertility	Esophagus, Pancreas, Kidney,
Polycystic Ovarian Syndrome (PCOS)	Prostate
Osteoarthritis	**Phlebitis**
Skin problems	**Gout**
Type-2 diabetes and metabolic syndrome	

Special note should be made of the relationship between type-2 diabetes and obesity. In fact, we have coined a new term for this disease. It is called "diabesity." *Isn't that great! We are creating new diseases, as if there aren't enough already.*

As the "terrorists" increase, the "hostile takeover" worsens. All of this happens through a process called chronic, low-grade, or "silent" inflammation. This kind of inflammation is not like the "screaming pain" you get from acute inflammation from a burn, cut, arthritis, or injury but is below the threshold of pain. Just because you don't feel the inflammation doesn't mean that it doesn't exist. It raises its ugly head in the form of heart attacks, strokes, loss of limbs, blindness, infections, and kidney failure.

Prior to the diabetes becoming a problem, another condition occurs. It is called **metabolic syndrome** or **insulin resistant syndrome**—IRS (it's like the IRS: it taxes you to death before it kills you).

To best understand how the metabolic syndrome works, you need to understand insulin. Insulin is a hormone secreted by the pancreas that is like a key that unlocks the door of a cell and lets blood sugar (glucose) into the cell. Blood sugar travels in the bloodstream and rises when we eat. Too much sugar in the blood causes diabetes, so the body uses insulin to get the sugar from the bloodstream into the cells, where it can be burned for energy. When someone gains too much weight, the key to the lock on the cell doesn't work as well, and it takes much more insulin to get the same amount of sugar into the cell. This is called insulin resistance and leads to the metabolic syndrome.

The blood sugar eventually returns to a normal level after large amounts of insulin override the system, but all of that excess insulin ends up hanging around in your blood, causing trouble. **Insulin is a storage enzyme that prevents you from breaking down fat and losing weight.** (Because of high insulin levels, you can almost look at a donut and gain five pounds.) In addition, excess insulin increases your appetite and contributes to hardening of the arteries by aggravating inflammation and free radical damage.

After a period of time, your pancreas no longer can produce the excess insulin that controls blood sugar, and levels start to increase, giving rise to type 2 diabetes. Then the "fun" begins with all the medical conditions associated with diabetes.

Even though diabetes is a problem in itself, the final common pathway for devastating problems is artery disease, especially in the heart. Diabetes leads to heart disease and strokes, which are the diseases that kill most diabetics. We lose a lot of wonderful people each year from these diseases, but the good news is they can potentially be prevented.

Metabolic syndrome has five criteria associated with it, and you only need three of them to make the diagnosis. Some require blood testing, but the first one can be done at home with a tape measure and is probably one of the best ways to make the diagnosis without blood work. Do you recognize it?

Metabolic Syndrome Criteria[6]

- Waist circumference: $\geq$ 40" for men and $\geq$35" for women (Caucasian)
  $\geq$ 35" for men and $\geq$31" for women (Asian)
- Blood pressure: $\geq$ 130/85 mm Hg
- HDL cholesterol: $\leq$ 40 mg/dl for men and $\leq$50 mg/dl for women
- Fasting blood sugar: > 110 mg/dl (new data suggests 100 mg/dl)
- Triglycerides: $\geq$ 150 mg/dl

Since the metabolic syndrome is a forerunner of type 2 diabetes, you should have your doctor check you for it by doing a blood test for insulin levels.

Metabolic syndrome is contributing to the "hostile takeover" by storing all the calories you eat and not allowing your body to burn fat. In addition, it increases your appetite and fuels chronic inflammation. Metabolic syndrome precedes type 2 diabetes by about eight to ten years.

It is interesting to note that 80–85 percent of diabetic subjects in North America and Europe have metabolic syndrome. However, most subjects with metabolic syndrome do not have diabetes. Metabolic syndrome predicts the development of type 2 diabetes and heart disease, and most importantly most people with metabolic syndrome are obese. See Figure I-4 of the Nurse's Health Study below to see just how closely diabetes follows obesity.

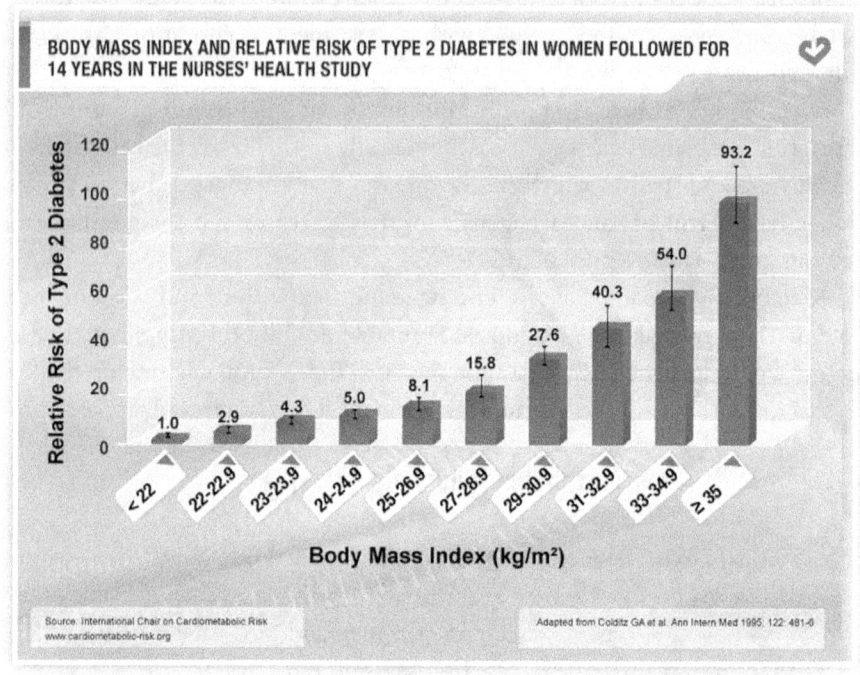

Figure I-4

Studies tell us that the prevalence of metabolic syndrome in the general public is 24 percent, but this is not a useful number since the prevalence of metabolic syndrome increases with age. It might be more useful to suggest that the prevalence of metabolic syndrome is the individual's age minus twenty. For example, if you are fifty years old, fifty minus twenty gives you thirty, or 30 percent of people fifty years of age have metabolic syndrome.[7] *That can really make birthdays scary.*

Enough said about medical conditions. Next we need to explore the deep recesses of emotion and our brains to discover what behaviors may be causing this epidemic of obesity.

CHAPTER 2

Behavioral Causes of Obesity

"It's too late for me, save yourself!" This seems to be the battle cry of too many people struggling with weight issues. Is that you?

As you can see, this quote has nothing to do with diet, exercise, medication, surgery, supplements, or gimmicks. It has everything to do with your attitude and behavior. This may sound simple, but it is a very complex process.

To become successful long term, you must change your behavior, and to do so you must first assume responsibility for your actions. This is well illustrated in a quote from Martin E. P. Seligman, PhD, in his book *Learned Optimism*:[8]

> Most assuredly we want people to own up to the messes they make, to be responsible for their actions. Certain psychological doctrines have damaged our society by helping to erode personal responsibility: Evil is mislabeled insanity; bad manners are shucked off as neurosis; "successfully

treated" patients evade their duty to their families because it does not bring them personal fulfillment.

The Promised Land

As we look at history, specifically that of the Israelites during their days of slavery in Egypt, we can learn a great deal about ourselves. Moses led the Israelites out of Egypt, but unfortunately (or fortunately), they took a forty-year detour through the wilderness before arriving at their destination. So, what does that have to do with weight loss? Everything!

Just look at the classic lyrics from the Eagles' song "Already Gone," which gives us our first clue.

> *Well, I know it wasn't you who held me down.*
> *Heaven knows it wasn't you who set me free.*
> *So often times it happens that we live our lives in chains,*
> *and we never even know we have the key.*

Often we look outside ourselves for the answers to why we are not successful. Our happiness, success, failures, etc., seem to stem from the external world. "If only" is our battle cry. *"If only he or she would treat me right, then I would be thin." "If only my circumstances were different, I wouldn't binge." "If only I were rich, then my troubles would go away."* And it goes on and on and on.

As individuals, we need to take a closer look at ourselves and discover why we are in this situation—this slavery. What happened to bring us to this point? Our solution is *"If only I could leave the slavery and get to the Promised Land, all would be well."* Does that work? For example, how many times have we heard of someone winning millions in the lottery only to be broke a few short years later? What is missing in this rag-to-riches story?

From a sermon given by Dr. Jack Stephenson of Anona United Methodist Church in Largo, Florida, we get an answer. The missing link is the wandering through the wilderness. You might ask, "Why would someone want to wander in the wilderness after just being freed from slavery?" Very simply, to learn and understand what caused them to be in slavery in the first place. We learn and grow to be successful in the Promised Land. If we arrive without improving, we are destined to make the same mistakes we made before. Think of how many people get "free" from the slavery of obesity only to regain their weight again and return to bondage. They forgot to go through the wilderness, such as a two- or three-year maintenance program, where they learn to grow and find their "key." You might say they went from rags to riches to rags" again.

Often, we have the key to our success but never seem to find it because it is the LAST thing we want to face—Lonely, Angry, Sad, Tired. These are some key reasons why you might sabotage your weight-loss success and stay stuck in shackles. There is a great Promised Land of health, freedom, happiness, and success if you will follow the path. Go through the wilderness of taking responsibility, learning, practicing, confronting, changing, and using your key to success that sets you free.

Follow the journey out of slavery into the wilderness. It will prepare you for what is to come—the Promised Land of authentic happiness and joy, not to mention a lean, mean, fat-burning machine.

Looking for True Happiness

Too many times we feel that there is a short-cut to happiness and joy. All we need to do is have as many pleasures in your life as possible. We are living the "good life," enjoying things like fine dining, chocolate, flowers, eating, a massage, eating, fine wine, eating, a good movie, eating, a new car, ice cream, pizza, or new clothes—not to mention eating. We are students of "happiology," more correctly termed "hedonics," which is the science of how we feel from moment to moment. A hedonist wants as many good moments and as few bad moments as possible in life.[9]

So, do the pleasures of life bring us true and authentic happiness? A great quote from the book *Authentic Happiness* by Martin Seligman, PhD, says it quite well:

> The belief that we can rely on shortcuts to happiness, joy, rapture, comfort, and ecstasy rather than be entitled to these feelings by the exercise of personal strengths and virtues leads to legions of people who in the middle of great wealth are starving spiritually. Positive emotions alienated from the exercise of character lead to emptiness, to inauthenticity, to depression, and as we age, to the gnawing realization that we are fidgeting until we die.[10]

Happiness is a combination of two states, pleasures and gratifications.

Pleasures are delights that have strong sensory and emotional components. They are the "raw feelings" of ecstasy, thrills, orgasm, exuberance, and comfort. They are the bodily delights. However, it is not easy to build your life around them, because they are all just momentary and require no thinking. They fade very rapidly once you become accustomed to them (habituation). The pleasure of the second bite of a fine chocolate ice cream is less than half the first. Pleasures work better if we spread them out over time and intermittently "get our fix."

Gratifications, on the other hand, are activities that we like doing but don't necessarily have the "raw feelings" accompanying them. Gratifications engage us fully, and we become immersed in them to the extent that time stands still. Examples are acts of kindness, dancing, reading a good book, rock-climbing, a hobby, learning to play a sport, playing an instrument, helping at the homeless shelter, making a new friend, raising children, worshiping God, or having a great conversation. "The gratifications last longer than the pleasures, they involve quite a lot of thinking and interpretation, they do not habituate easily, and they are undergirded by our strengths and virtues," according to Dr. Seligman.

"Pleasure marks the achievement of biological satiation, whereas gratification marks the achievement of psychological growth." This was illustrated in a study of teenagers who were pleasure or "mall" kids; they hung out at malls and watched TV a lot. On the other hand gratification kids had hobbies, they engaged in sports, and they spent a lot of time on homework.

Another quote from Dr. Seligman's book states it so well.

> Pleasure is a powerful source of motivation, but it does not produce change; it is a conservative force that makes us want to satisfy existing needs, achieve comfort and relaxation...Enjoyment [gratification] on the other hand is not always pleasant, and it can be utterly stressful at times. A mountain climber may be close to freezing, utterly exhausted in danger of falling into a bottomless crevasse, yet he wouldn't want to be anywhere else. Sipping a cocktail under a palm tree at the edge of the turquoise ocean is nice, but it just doesn't compare to the exhilaration he feels on the freezing ridge.[11]

So it is with having a healthy weight. It becomes a gratification and not a pleasure. It becomes the "stuff" of what your life is made—your strengths and virtues. To get there you must understand what motivates all behavior and how to gain pleasure in your gratifications. There are certain things you need to know.

Let's begin!

Stages of Behavioral Change

To find your "key" and free yourself from bondage, you must understand behavior and how it changes. James O. Prochaska, PhD, developed a useful model for understanding how people change. It is called the Stages of Behavioral Change.[12] These stages are:

- **Pre-contemplation**: People are unaware of the problem behavior or have no plans to change in the foreseeable future, usually measured as the next six months.
- **Contemplation**: People acknowledge the problem and are considering changing. Clinicians often make the mistake of thinking that the person is ready to change in this stage, but that is not the case. They are still only thinking about changing.
- **Preparation**: People are intending to take action in the immediate future. They are on the verge and making preparations to take action.
- **Action**: People have made specific overt modifications in their lifestyles. They make the move and implement the plan.
- **Maintenance**: People are struggling to prevent relapse, a stage which is estimated to last "from six months to about five years." A lapse is one slipup, a relapse is two or more, and a collapse is back to square one.
- **Termination**: The individuals have zero temptation and 100 percent own the new behavior. They are sure they will not return to their old, unhealthy habits as a way of coping with life.

Each behavior you want to change (like exercising more, eating less, or losing weight) is at one of the stages of change. You may be at pre-contemplation on exercise (never even gave it a thought) but at preparation for losing weight.

Pain and Pleasure of Changing

Now that you have an understanding about the stages of change, the next question is "How do I change?" You have to get leverage on yourself so that you *want* to change, and that comes from understanding Dr. Sigmund Freud's "pain and pleasure" principles. People will do anything to avoid pain and everything to gain pleasure. This is psychologist Kurt Lewin's approach-avoidance concept, which is taught in psychology 101.

Pick a behavior that you want to change. Let's say, for example, that you want to lose thirty-five pounds. Your goal is to be thirty-five pounds thinner in six months. Or you can substitute your own personal goal. Remember the Five Ps of goal setting:[13]

- Personal
- Positive
- Precise
- Present
- Possible

My goal is:

> **"Goals are the breakfast of champions."**
> **They are a dream with a time line.**
> —Denis Waitley, *The Psychology of Winning*

Steven K. Scott, co-founder of American Telecast Corporation, states: "The Law of Dream Conversion: Convert dreams into goals, goals into tasks, and tasks into steps."[14]

Next, insert your written goal in the blank spaces below, and answer these four questions.

What is the pain of _____?

What is the pleasure of _____?

What is the pain of NOT _____?

What is the pleasure of NOT _____?

Write each question at the top of separate pieces of paper. Start answering each question by writing down your answers below it. The first few answers will be obvious and simple. For example, the pleasure of being thirty-five pounds thinner in six months might be "I will look good in clothes." Write that answer on the paper and go to the next answer.

Once you write an answer, you cannot use it again. Soon you will get to what really motivates or "bothers" you. What is really enslaving you? That is what you want to know and face. Keep going. Remember, this list is for your eyes only.

What you may discover is that you need professional help. That is OK. Get it!

The purpose of this exercise is to gain insight into your behavior. **You do things for your reasons and no one else's.** You might as well know what those reasons are, because that gets you "ready, willing, and able" to change."

Ready, Willing, and Able

From the book *Motivational Interviewing*[15] comes a very powerful technique in changing behavior. It is based on the old colloquialism called "ready, willing, and able." These are three critical components of motivation.

1. **Ready** has to do with your relative priorities: *"I want to, but not now."* Not being ready can stop everything in its tracks. The mindset of not being ready has also become the symbol of self-deception: *"I'll change tomorrow."*
2. **Willing** is your perceived importance of changing. It is the discrepancy between what is happening now (status quo) and what you value in the future (goals). As long as your present situation is within desired limits, no change will occur. Willingness is the **commitment** to change.
3. **Able** concerns itself with how optimistic or pessimistic you are that you can change. It's the *"I wish I could"* mindset. "Able" is the **confidence** to change.

When a situation is important enough, people believe that a change will work, and that they can do it. Then they will change. On the other hand, when people see no way of changing, they will reduce their discomfort level by shifting their thought processes to a "defensive" mode. The classic defense mechanisms are an example of this. They will use denial (*"It's not really so bad"*), rationalization (*"I didn't want it anyway"*), and projection (*"It's not my problem, it's theirs"*).

People don't like change, but this can be a key to success if you recognize it for what it is—an **opportunity**. If you find yourself being resistant, you are probably following an old script that you have played many times before. This is the expected role or response for you to make. Your lines are predictable, and you have rehearsed and perfected them over the years. [10, 15]

To view resistance as a character flaw is a sad mistake because it lies at the very heart of change. It arises from your many motives and struggles, and it foreshadows your future actions. You just need to know how to change your sails in the winds of resistance in order to arrive at a new and exciting port. This can be accomplished by being committed and confident.[16]

So how do we put this together and make it happen? Simple! Answer the following three questions.

Commitment and Confidence Scale[17]

Using a scale from 0 to 10 where 0 is "no interest" and 10 is "let's do it yesterday," answer the following questions.

How ready are you to act?
Score:_____

How willing or committed are you to change?
Score:_____

How able or confident are you in being able to accomplish this goal?
Score:_____

Now look at your scores. Why is your score what it is and not 0? What got you to that point? What has to happen to raise the score two or three more points?

By answering these three simple questions, you can assess your level of readiness and make a better prediction of your success.

Suppose that you scored 7 or 8 on committed or willing but only a 2 or 3 on confidence or able. This means that you are ready and willing but don't think that you can do it. You lack confidence and might be remembering past failures.

Since in the example your score for confidence was at least 2 or 3 and not 0, you have some reason to believe that you can be successful. Something is giving you hope. What has to happen to raise your confidence just two more points? Remember the Law of Dream Conversion?[18] What "tasks" need to be accomplished to convert them into "steps," and those "steps" into "goals?"

Do the same thing with your ready and willing scores. How is your commitment level? What will it take to raise it two more points?

Remember: "It is hard by the yard, but a cinch by the inch."

Habit of Success

Armed with the tools you now possess, it is time to act. You want to be successful, and you want success to become a habit.

Remember the great words of the English poet and playwright John Dryden:

"We first make our habits, and then our habits make us."

What habits have you made? Are you following the habits of a tribe you no longer belong to? It is now time to evaluate everything. It is the time to create and incorporate only the habits of success.

From famed motivational speaker Denis Waitley, we learn that it takes a month to create a new habit and one to two years to make it permanent. So, when you start to develop a new habit and have a lapse or mess up, realize that this is normal. It's obvious that you will "screw up" during something that takes you two years. "We are only human," as singer Billy Joel says, and we need our "second wind." **The tragedy is not in messing up but in quitting.** As Americans, we don't like quitters. We love the "hero" who gets up after being knocked down and fights back like Rocky Balboa in the movie *Rocky*.

In your quest to develop more proactive habits, many obstacles will occur. Your job is to push through using the knowledge that you have acquired and not quit. Understanding what is important and "empowers" you is crucial. Take the information that you have learned and *use* it. Understand your personal "pain and pleasure" and what makes you "ready, willing, and able" to succeed. Tap into your resources of friends, support groups, church, professionals, education, and family.

Remember, just thinking that the pleasures of life will get you through is a fallacy. They become your bondage and hold you captive. Gratifications, using your strengths and virtues. are the key that will set you free to enjoy life more as a thinner, healthier, more gratified you.

Be a big "loser" and not a quitter.

Believe me, I wouldn't say this if I hadn't been there myself.

As Mark Twain said, "Twenty years from now you will be more disappointed by the things you didn't do than by the ones you did. So, throw off the bowlines. Sail away from safe harbor. Catch the trade winds in your sails. Explore. Dream. Discover."

CHAPTER 3

Psychological Barriers to Successful Weight Loss

To be a "loser" in weight loss, you must understand some of the psychological barriers that prevent you from reaching your goals. **Just like we discussed with obesity, these are diseases and not character flaws.** Many require professional medical or psychiatric help. The purpose of this chapter is to make you aware.

Once again, these psychological problems are the LAST thing you want to be—Lonely, Angry, Sad, and Tired. They are the "little foxes that spoil the vines." When you are experiencing these feelings, you are very vulnerable and might start thinking, *"To heck with it, I'm going to eat what I want." "Forget this program, it doesn't work." "It's too late for me. Save yourself!"* The excuses begin.

All of these are the battle cry of "learned helplessness." From Dr. Seligman we learn:

Learned helplessness is the giving-up reaction, the quitting response that follows from the belief that whatever you do doesn't matter. *Explanatory style* is the manner in which you habitually explain to yourself why events happen. It is the great modulator of learned helplessness. An optimistic explanatory style stops helplessness, whereas a pessimistic explanatory style spreads helplessness. Your way of explaining events to yourself determines how helpless you can become, or how energized, when you encounter the everyday setbacks as well as momentous defeats. I think of your explanatory style as reflecting "the word in your heart."[19]

So when learned helplessness raises its ugly head and the excuses begin, do you want comfort, like "comfort foods?"

"Comfort foods" are also known as "momma foods," which are "soft, chewy, moist, warm, creamy, smooth and sweet." If you are in the party mood then "icy, spicy, tingly, tangy, crunchy, crackly, and salty" foods will do. These are great descriptions from Ralph Carson, PhD, RD.[20] Let's start moving away from a victim mentality, or learned helplessness, by changing our thinking pattern. These are profound words by Dr. Tom Massey:

> Justice appears in the world through the process of cause and effect, not by the action of a Divine Judge intent on punishing us for the mistakes we make. We are not punished for our mistakes—but *by* them. Each of us must assume responsibility for our own actions.[21]

To become responsible for your own actions and break from the ruts in your life of mediocrity, conventional wisdom, and group thinking, you must have a plan and the mental tools to accomplish it. You need to become the CEO of your own life.

As CEO, your first duty is to assume responsibility. You want to change, but you will not change unless you assume responsibility. You must clean up your own mess and be accountable to yourself and others. **The crime is not in having a weight problem but in not doing something about it.**

In his book *The Seven Habits of Highly Effective People*, Steven Covey defines responsibility as "response-ability." He says:

> Highly proactive people recognize responsibility. They do not blame circumstances, conditions, or conditioning for their behavior. Their

behavior is a product of their own conscious choice based on values, rather than a product of their conditions, based on feeling.[22]

You must take personal control of your life, which by definition means "the ability to change things by voluntary actions." Personal control or empowerment is the opposite of helplessness. **Take charge and empower your life.**

The great news about learned helplessness is that you can change. Notice the word "learned." Something learned can be unlearned. You need to create a new habit of success. This book is about change and giving you the tools needed to succeed, but only *you* can do it.

The first place to start is getting rid of your old excuses. These are "failure talk" and are no longer part of your vocabulary. In his book *Excuses Begone!* Dr. Wayne W. Dyer states: "In my role as a counselor, teacher, and parent, I've heard many reasons that people use to explain an unhappy existence…and almost all of them inevitably fall into one huge category, which I call 'Excuses.'"[23]

Just think of the excuses we can use. Here is a list from Dr. Dyer:

1. It will be difficult.
2. It will take a long time.
3. There will be family drama.
4. It's not my nature.
5. I can't afford it.
6. No one will help me.
7. It will be risky.
8. It has never happened before.
9. I'm not strong enough.
10. I'm not smart enough.
11. I'm too old (or not old enough).
12. The rules won't let me.
13. It's too big.
14. I don't have the energy.
15. It's my personal family history.
16. I'm too busy.
17. I'm too scared.

Do any sound familiar? You might need to revisit the previous chapter on how to gain leverage on yourself and make changes, and start with a good attitude.

Now let's shift our thinking to behavioral problems that might require professional help. **Again, these are diseases that can be treated.** As we said, the shame is not in having the problem but in not getting the proper help.

Get ED Out of Your Head[24]

ED can definitely get into your head and cause problems, but who is ED?

ED is an acronym for Eating Disorders. Eating disorders are a disease or group of conditions characterized by abnormal eating habits that may involve excessive or insufficient food intake to the detriment of an individual's physical and emotional health. ED is thought to affect primarily females (five to ten million in the US) but affects males as well (one million in the US).[25]

The most common eating disorders are Eating Disorder Not Otherwise Stated (EDNOS—a wastebasket term for many types of disorders), Binge Eating Disorder (BED), Bulimia Nervosa (BN), and Anorexia Nervosa (AN).

Remember that many people suffering with ED were physically, mentally, or sexually abused as a child or adult. Treatments are available for these disorders, but professional help is necessary to treat them.

Binge Eating Disorder (BED)

Binge Eating Disorder, also known as Compulsive Eating Disorder, is the most common ED in the United States, affecting 3.5 percent of females and 2 percent of males, and **is prevalent in up to 30 percent of those seeking treatment in a weight-loss clinic.** Be aware!

A "binge" is defined as eating a large amount of food (up to ten thousand calories) in a short period of time (less than two hours) and feeling out of control. Snacking is not binging.

The criteria for BED includes binging at least two times per week for six months, marked distress, guilty feelings, depressed, hiding food, and lack of control. There is no purging or compensatory action (vomiting, water pills, laxatives, or excessive exercise).

Bulimia Nervosa (BN)

Ninety percent of people suffering with Bulimia Nervosa are women. In addition, 80 percent are normal weight, 10 percent are below weight, and 10 percent are overweight. These are the "shoppers" to weight-loss clinics.

People with BN suffer from the delusion that no matter how many compliments they receive, their body is not attractive enough. The definition of a BN includes binging at least two times per week for three months. In addition, 80 to 90 percent purge (finger down throat to induce vomiting, laxative abuse, water pill abuse, enemas, or obsessive exercise).

Anorexia Nervosa (AN)

With AN, 90 percent are females usually from a higher socioeconomic status, and many come from a dysfunctional family setting.

AN is defined as a refusal to maintain minimal body weight (BMI~16) along with an intense fear of gaining weight. People who suffer from this disorder have a distorted body image.

Nocturnal Sleep-Related Eating Disorder (NSRED)

NSRED should be briefly mentioned. Even though it is primarily a sleep disorder, overeating is part of it. People suffering from this disorder are totally unaware that they are eating. They awaken in the morning to find empty food wrappers and crumbs, but they have no recollection of consuming this food.

This disorder is a combination of eating disorder and sleep disorder. Contrast this to Nocturnal Eating Disorder, which is a disorder where a person is totally aware of overeating at night, but cannot help it. Also, this disorder can occur in people taking certain sleep medications.

Mood Disorders

Depression is the disease state most associatied with mood disorders. The common definition is a state of sadness when you lose something of importance. The psychiatric definition is "an abnormal mood akin to the sadness, unhappiness, and misery of everyday experience along with the inability to experience pleasure."[26]

Mood disorder victims experience a depressed mood (may be irritability in children and adolescents), marked diminished interest or pleasure, insomnia, fatigue, feelings of worthlessness, inappropriate guilt, diminished ability to think or concentrate, and recurrent thoughts of death.

There is a 15 percent lifetime prevalence of depression in the general population. The most worrisome problem is the **15 percent risk of suicide among depressed patients.** As with all of these disorders, seek professional help.

Generalized Anxiety Disorders

Anxiety is defined as a state of continual apprehension in which a person experiences excessive worry, irritability, inability to relax, forgetfulness, and "stress eating."

There is a 5 percent lifetime prevalence of this disorder, and it can be associated with drug abuse and depression.

Obsessive Compulsive Disorder

Obsessive–compulsive disorder (OCD) one of the most common mental disorders in the US. One in fifty American adults has OCD. People who suffer from OCD experience intrusive thoughts that produce anxiety, and often feel compelled to perform repetitive behaviors in order to reduce their anxiety. Symptoms include the following:

- Repetitive hand washing
- Hoarding
- Preoccupation with sexual or aggressive impulses
- Preoccupation with particular religious beliefs
- Aversion to odd numbers
- Nervous habits, such as opening and closing a door a certain number of times before entering or leaving a room.

These symptoms can be so powerful that they impact a person's social and financial well-being.

Attention Deficit Hyperactivity Disorder (ADHD)

There is a lifetime prevalence of this disorder of 8 percent. Many adults suffered with it in childhood. Fortunately, some children can out grow it.

ADHD is defined as a disorder in which a person is very impulsive and makes no plans. He or she has trouble completing tasks and is distracted easily. People with ADHD seem not to listen and have a poor sense of time and time management.

A characteristic that fools other people is the ADHD person's ability to concentrate. If people with ADHD are very interested in something, they have extreme focus and concentration. Most of the time, they have a lack of concentration. That is why obesity treatment does not work for many.

Personality Disorders

Personality disorders, formerly referred to as character disorders, are a class of personality types and behaviors that the American Psychiatric Association (APA) defines as "an enduring pattern of inner experience and behavior that deviates markedly from the expectations of the culture of the individual who exhibits it…is pervasive and inflexible (unlikely to change), is stable over time, and leads to distress in…relationships." In fact, "The very definition of a personality disorder is that it causes distress for both the person who has the disorder and those who interact with them."[27]

The onset of these patterns of behavior can typically be traced back to late adolescence and the beginning of adulthood and, in rarer instances, childhood. It is therefore unlikely that a diagnosis of personality disorder will be appropriate before the age of sixteen or seventeen years.

There are several types of personality disorders. To name a few:

- **Paranoid**: characterized by irrational suspicions and mistrust of others.
- **Schizoid**: lack of interest in social relationships; seeing no point in sharing time with others.
- **Histrionic**: pervasive attention-seeking behavior including inappropriate sexual seductiveness and shallow or exaggerated emotions.
- **Borderline**: extreme "black and white" thinking; instability in relationships, self-image, identity, and behavior.
- **Narcissistic**: a pervasive pattern of grandiosity, need for admiration, and a lack of empathy for others.
- **Passive-Aggressive**: a pattern of negative attitudes and passive resistance in interpersonal situations.

If you or someone you know shows signs and symptoms of any of these disorders, seek professional help. Those who suffer from them can only be treated by a trained professional. Always remember that they are disorders of the brain and not character flaws. Treat others and yourself compassionately.

Now let's move on to our stomachs and talk about food.

CHAPTER 4

The Simple Facts of Nutrition

Guess what? Did you know that you need food to function?

Isn't that amazing? Food provides our bodies with the energy and nutrients to survive and perform. So, if that is so "amazing," why do we put the wrong kinds of food in our bodies and expect it to function at peak performance? That doesn't make sense. Why not just use the "good stuff" in the first place?

To be able to use the "good stuff," you need to understand six types of nutrients: carbohydrates, fats, proteins, vitamins and minerals, antioxidants, and water.

We use these nutrients to provide us with energy to grow, repair our cells and organs, and control our body's functions. All of these nutrients are important for our body to function at its peak. If you lack any of these nutrients, you will not function at your best. No wonder with the many weight-management programs out there, which restrict certain nutrients or forget to add them, we are gaining weight and facing more and more chronic diseases. *That only makes job security for physicians.*

Let's examine each of the types of nutrients and how they impact our bodies in order to improve our nutritional decisions. We will divide them into macronutrients, which are carbohydrates, protein, and fats; and micronutrients, which are vitamins, minerals, and water.

So, it is back to school—Nutrition 101.

Carbohydrates

Carbohydrates or "carbs" are the major source of fuel for the body. Examples of carbohydrates are fruits, vegetables, legumes, beans, and grain products. A special class of carbs is starches. These include sugar, potatoes, rice, pasta, bread, bagels, donuts, and flour.

Carbohydrates are made up of the elements carbon, hydrogen, and oxygen, and they break down into waste products of water and carbon dioxide. We get rid of the carbon dioxide through our lungs and the excess water through sweating and the kidneys.

We can divide carbohydrates into simple and complex. The major difference is that complex carbohydrates have fiber, and because of the fiber it takes the body longer to digest these carbohydrates, so they enter the bloodstream slower. This in turn doesn't raise the blood sugars too quickly, making them a better dietary choice.

Sugars

The simple sugars with only one single sugar molecule (monosaccharides) are glucose (blood sugar), fructose (fruit sugar), and galactose. If you made a new sugar molecule by chemically mixing glucose and fructose, you would have sucrose (table sugar). If you mixed glucose and galactose, you would have lactose (milk sugar). If you mixed glucose and glucose, you would get maltose (malt sugar).

Many adults lack the enzyme lactase that breaks down lactose or milk sugar for digestion. When they drink milk, the lactose can cause bloating, cramps, and diarrhea. This is called lactose intolerance. Sometimes buying the enzyme lactase at a health-food store can help this condition.

Starches

Complex carbohydrates are broken into two categories, digestible (starches) and indigestible (fiber).

Starches are the major carbohydrate in our diets and are found in potatoes, beans, breads, pasta, and rice. Your body first stores these carbohydrates in the muscle and liver cells in long strings of glucose (like G-G-G-G-G-G) called glycogen (*you might even call it a G-string*) and releases them into the bloodstream as needed for quick energy. If you consume too many calories from carbohydrates, these excess carbohydrates are converted into fat and stored you know where.

Sugar alcohols like xylitol, sorbitol, erythrithol, etc., are similar to sucrose and taste sweet, but they cannot be digested. They are used for many sugar-free products. In addition, they do not promote tooth decay like sugar, but consuming too much of them can cause cramps and diarrhea.

Let's take a moment and discuss another alcohol—ethanol, or booze. You know beer, wine, and liquor, the three main food groups. Alcohol has seven calories per gram, while proteins and carbohydrates only have four calories per gram. Fat has nine calories per gram. Alcohol is a calorie-dense food, but that is not the main problem. When you drink alcohol, it is not used like carbohydrates for instant energy, but instead it is *first stored as fat*. To get the energy from alcohol, it first must be stored and then *later* released and burned. This is one of the problems with drinking too much alcohol, it gets stored, guess where (beer belly)? In addition there is always a potential for over consumption and alcoholism. Be careful and only drink responsibly.

Fiber

Fiber is further divided into insoluble and soluble.

Examples of insoluble fiber are wheat bran, wheat products, and brown rice. Insoluble fiber acts like a scrub brush on the inside of the intestines and colon and helps do house cleaning. Insoluble fiber is Mother Nature's "colon cleanser."

Soluble types of fiber are found in apples, bananas, oranges, carrots, barley, oats, and kidney beans. Other types of soluble fiber are gum arabic, guar gum, locus bean gum, and pectin. Soluble fiber can bind with fats and cholesterol in the diet and decrease or slow their absorption into the bloodstream. For people with cholesterol problems, this can be very beneficial.

Fibers are undigested as they pass through the gut and help form the bulk of the stool. Sometimes colon bacteria can partially digest the fiber, causing intestinal gas. In addition, fiber slows the stomach from emptying so quickly and increases the feeling of fullness (satiety). This slows down the absorption of other carbohydrates and creates a smooth release of sugar into the bloodstream from the gut. The American Dietetic Association (ADA) recommends twenty to thirty-five grams of fiber a day. Remember to slowly start increasing your fiber intake, and you may need over-the-counter products for gas and cramps like Bean-O, Gas-X, etc.

Glycemic Index

Another consideration when examining carbohydrates is glycemic index (GI). The GI is defined as how high and how quickly blood sugar rises after eating a specific carbohydrate. The area under the curve increases, for you science "geeks." The higher the GI measurement, the more like sugar a carbohydrate is. For instance, table sugar causes a quick response so it has a high GI. Oatmeal, on the other hand, because of the fiber has a much slower response; therefore, its GI is low.

The GI of a particular meal can be changed by adding fat and protein to lower the GI. If you are eating white bread and jelly, you will have a high GI. By adding some peanut butter or cottage cheese to the snack, you will slow down absorption and therefore lower the GI of the meal.

Glycemic index is very important when dealing with diabetes and metabolic syndrome. When you have a fast spike in your blood sugar, you get an equally fast and sometimes too high of a spike of insulin. Remember, insulin is the hormone from the pancreas that acts like a key to open the door to the cells and allow the sugar from the bloodstream to enter. Obesity can cause the cells of the body to be insulin resistant, so it takes a great deal more insulin to do the same job.

This excess insulin causes trouble by increasing your appetite, preventing fat cells from releasing fat, storing most of the calories that you eat, aggravating hardening of the arteries (atherosclerosis), and leading to the metabolic syndrome (MS), also known as the insulin resistant syndrome. Understanding MS is important because it leads to type-2 diabetes, but it can be controlled and possibly prevented.

In addition, exaggerated spikes in blood sugar after a high-GI meal generate excess free radicals that can trigger a biochemical tsunami resulting in inflammation that leads to degenerative diseases like diabetes, Alzheimer's dementia, heart disease, and obesity. This is proven by the fact that recent studies have shown that about one-third of American adults and two-thirds of heart patients have abnormal blood sugar problems without yet being considered a diabetic.[28]

Another measurement is called the glycemic load (GL). You simply take the GI and multiply it by the serving size. This is a more accurate measurement, because some foods, like carrots, have a high GI but when multiplied by serving size are OK. They don't have such an influence on insulin spikes.

Your diet needs to contain complex carbohydrates and lower GI or GL foods. This possibly helps prevent metabolic syndrome, obesity, and type 2 diabetes.

Fats and Oils

Lipids or fats are the next food source we need to discuss. They are great sources of energy (nine calories/gram), and they give food a moist and juicy taste. Foods would taste dry without fats. (What do you think makes a great burger?) In addition, our bodies need good fats to live and function. The body needs fats to form your organs, cell membranes, eyes, immune system, brain, hormones, and help in the healing of wounds.

Fats in your diet can be divided into saturated and unsaturated. Unsaturated fats are further subdivided into monounsaturated or polyunsaturated fatty acids (PUFA). PUFA are again further subdivided into omega-3 or omega-6 fatty acids. (Are you thoroughly confused over the different forms of grease?)

Saturated fats are solids at room temperature and are considered hard fats. This quality is what causes them to stick to the inner lining of arteries and promote hardening of the arteries (atherosclerosis), which leads to heart attacks. Examples of saturated fats are butter, margarine, lard, milk fat, and most animal fats.

Along with saturated fats, we need to discuss trans fats. In order to improve profit margins and maintain the texture in food, the food industry created trans fats. Trans fats increase LDL cholesterol (bad—L is Lousy and you want it Low) and decrease HDL cholesterol (good—H is Healthy and you want it High), which promotes heart disease. Luckily the government has stepped in and restricted the use of trans fats in our foods. Because deep-frying causes trans fats to form, you need to be careful of hidden trans fats in foods like french fries or deep-fried foods. *Oops!*

Next we have monounsaturated fats like canola and olive oil. This is also known as an omega-9 fatty acid and promotes good health when consumed in moderation. However, be careful to not fry food in olive oil, since high temperatures change its configuration.

The polyunsaturated fats (PUFA) are omega-6 and omega-3 fats. Examples of omega-6 fats are corn, soybean, sunflower, and safflower oils. Examples of omega-3 fatty acids are fish oils and flaxseed oil.

People consume about ten to twenty times more omega-6 oils than omega-3 oils. The ratio should be about one to one. In other words, we need to eat more fish and flaxseed oil and much less plant oils like corn, safflower, sunflower, and soybean.

Long-chain omega-3 fish oil has been shown to be good for the heart. Flaxseed is a short-chain omega-3 and has not shown to be as heart protective. When you consume short-chain flaxseed oil, only about 15 to 20 percent is converted to the heart protective long chain form. That doesn't mean flaxseed isn't good for you. It is. Just eat your cold-water fish or seafood.

Another lipid is cholesterol, but it is not a true fat. Cholesterol, though given a bad rap, is needed in forming many of the hormones in our body, like estrogen and testosterone. We need cholesterol but in the right form and amounts.

Fat is digested in the stomach and absorbed in the small intestines with the help of bile from the gall bladder.   When fat is absorbed from the gut into the bloodstream, proteins are attached to the fat to help cells identify what type of fat it is and where it is to be used (the protein is like a taxi that carries the passenger fat). Examples are HDL cholesterol (good cholesterol—H is *happy* and you want it *high*) and LDL cholesterol (bad cholesterol—L is *lousy* and you want it *low*).

HDL is produced in the liver and is the scavenger that picks up extra cholesterol from the body and helps eliminate it. It also helps prevent LDL from sticking to the blood vessel walls and causing hardening of the arteries. That is why it is called the good cholesterol and LDL is called the bad cholesterol.

Proteins

Proteins (Greek word for "ports"—to come first) are the next macronutrient. They are very important since they are vital for most all of our bodily functions and exist in every cell. They are involved in the regulation of our energy, fluid maintenance, blood clotting, hormones, and enzyme production, repairing and building of cells.

Unlike fat reserves and a smaller amount of carbohydrate reserves, there are no reserves of protein. Therefore, you need to consume protein daily. A person is capable of using twenty-five to thirty grams of protein at one feeding. Since cooked meat, fish, or fowl has seven grams of protein per ounce, a serving of four to five ounces is adequate per meal. Unfortunately, 65 percent of all protein is consumed after six thirty p.m. Your body cannot utilize it all at once, so the protein is broken down and made into fats and carbohydrates. That can create a protein deficiency in a well-fed person. The key is to spread your protein consumption throughout the day in snacks and meals.[29]

Proteins are composed of amino acids, and there are twenty-two amino acids that make up all proteins. Most of them are called nonessential because our body can make them from other amino acids. Nine are called essential amino acids, and that means that our bodies cannot make them. So they need to be consumed daily. We need particular amino acids in order to function: histidine, tryptophan, isoleucine, leucine lysine, methionine, phenylalanine, threonine, and valine.

Our foods provide a combination of essential and nonessential amino acids in different proportions. Complete or high-quality proteins provide all of the eight essential amino acids. Most plant proteins are low-quality or incomplete proteins because they are missing one or more of the eight essential amino acids. That is why vegans and vegetarians need to combine plant sources of protein in order to get all of the essential amino acids.

A major function of proteins in the body (albumin and globulins) is to maintain bodily fluids. These large proteins are in the bloodstream and help attract fluids from the tissues back into the blood vessels, preventing swollen tissues. If the proteins are low, you have swollen legs or edema. Proteins are also needed to maintain the acid-base balance, form hormones, boost the immune system, and sometimes are used for energy.

Vitamins and Minerals

A vitamin is an organic compound required as a nutrient in tiny amounts. It cannot be made in sufficient quantities by the body and must be obtained from the diet. Vitamins are needed to help make your body function.

Vitamins have diverse biochemical functions. Some have hormone-like functions as regulators of mineral metabolism (vitamin D) or regulators of cell and tissue growth and differentiation (vitamin A). Others function as antioxidants (vitamin E and sometimes vitamin C). The largest number of vitamins (B vitamins) functions as building blocks for enzymes.

There are two different types of vitamins—fat-soluble and water soluble. Fat-soluble vitamins (A, D, E, and K) dissolve in fat (cell membranes) and are not easily excreted from the body. Fat-soluble vitamins in large quantities can be toxic or poisonous. Water-soluble vitamins, on the other hand, dissolve in water and are easily excreted from the body. They need to be replaced on a regular basis.

Fat-Soluble Vitamins

Vitamin A (retinol) is needed especially for vision, healthy skin, bone growth, and for the immune system. It is found in liver, fish, fish oils, fortified milk, eggs, and dark green and yellow-orange vegetables and fruits like carrots, spinach, winter squash, sweet potatoes, broccoli, mangoes, cantaloupes, peaches, and apricots.

Vitamin D is produced when the sun converts a form of cholesterol into vitamin D in your skin. Being exposed to the sun on your arms and legs for about ten minutes a day can create up to twenty thousand IU of vitamin D. If you are taking a supplement, it is very important also to consume calcium and phosphorus with the vitamin D. Fatty fish like sardines and salmon, as well as fortified milk, are the main sources of vitamin D.

Vitamin E (tocopherol) is an antioxidant in cell membranes and plays a role in our immune system especially as we age. Vitamin E is mainly found in plant oils, many fruits, and wheat germ, but it is not found in animal fats.

Vitamin K is essential for blooding clotting and is found in many foods like cabbage and spinach. It is also produced by bacteria in our colon.

Water-Soluble Vitamins

Thiamin (vitamin B1) helps utilize carbohydrates and some of the amino acids. It keeps mucous membranes healthy and helps the nervous system, muscle function, and heart function. It is found in pork, sunflower seeds, legumes, watermelon, whole grains, and mushrooms. Beriberi is caused by lack of vitamin B1 with symptoms of anorexia, weight loss, apathy, numbness, and weakness. We see this problem often in alcoholics and more recently in some obese patients who have had gastric bypass surgery.

Riboflavin (vitamin B2) is needed for cells to function, especially in the respiratory and digestive systems. It is found in milk, mushrooms, and green leafy vegetables as well as cottage cheese.

Niacin (vitamin B3) is a major regulator of the body's chemical processes. It is the co-helper in two hundred metabolic pathways. You can get niacin from poultry, brewer's yeast, peanuts, soybeans, and tuna. Niacin deficiency leads to pellagra, or the three Ds: dementia, diarrhea, and dermatitis. It has also been used to decrease LDL cholesterol, increase HDL levels, and decrease triglycerides.

Panthothenic (vitamin B5) helps metabolize carbohydrates, proteins, and fats as well as synthesize various enzymes. It is found in meats, mushrooms, peanuts, broccoli, lobster, and whole-grain products.

Biotin (vitamin H) is used in forming fatty acids and helps keep sweat glands functional as well as nerves, skin, and hair. Egg yolks are a great source of biotin, yet raw egg whites block the absorption of biotin.

Pyridoxine (vitamin B6) is involved in many reactions in the body such as carbohydrate metabolism, boosting neurotransmitters, and immune support. A deficiency causes reduced protein synthesis, weakness, seborrhea dermatitis, anemia, convulsions, depression, and confusion.

Folic acid (vitamin B9) is vital for the development of red blood cells, energizing the nervous system and immune systems, and protein synthesis. Deficiency of this vitamin occurs with alcohol abuse and chemotherapy, leading to anemia, weakness, lack of energy, decreased appetites, and forgetfulness. You can get folic acid from dark green leafy vegetables.

Cyanocobalamin (vitamin B12) needs to come from animal sources. It is vital for most bodily functions. Many disease processes, interfere, with its absorption. It is stored in the liver, and lack of it causes pernicious anemia. Strict vegans and vegetarians may need to take B12 replacements, since it is not in their diet.

Ascorbic acid (vitamin C) is extremely important for our health. It cannot be made in the body and is used for connective tissue development, wound healing, helping with calcium absorption, and stimulating red blood cell and antioxidant production. It is found in fruits and vegetables. Lack of vitamin C in the diet causes scurvy, delayed healing, loss of teeth, bruising, increased infections, and weakness.

Minerals

A **mineral** is a naturally occurring solid chemical substance that has a characteristic chemical composition, a highly ordered atomic structure, and specific physical properties.

Minerals are very important to bodily maintenance and function, and at least sixteen are essential for good health.

Sodium is readily absorbed from the intestinal tract and is excreted in our urine. It is very important in maintaining fluids in the right compartments. Sodium is also important in the body's electrical system. Lack of sodium causes severe thirst and weakness. Too much sodium leads to severe swelling (edema) and high blood pressure (hypertension).

Potassium regulates our body's fluid balance, nerve conduction, and muscle contractions. It is so vital that with too little we die and with too much we die. Symptoms of low potassium (hypokalemia) include muscle cramps, heart arrhythmias, confusion, constipation, and severe weakness. We obtain potassium from fresh fruits and vegetables especially winter squash, orange juice, cantaloupe, and bananas. Water pills (diuretics) can cause a decrease in potassium.

Calcium is stored in the bones, but because bone is always being broken down, reabsorbed, and rebuilt, you need to constantly replenish calcium through diet. As we age, bone starts to lose calcium, resulting in osteoporosis. In addition, calcium is needed for blood clotting, muscle contraction, and for nerve conduction. Calcium is found in many dairy products and leafy green vegetables.

Phosphorus is another mineral needed for bone formation and teeth health. It helps regulate calcium levels, bone formation, and growth.

Magnesium is needed for nerve and muscle function, heart rhythm, bone development, and healthy teeth. It helps with the regulation of insulin, and a lack of it results in weakness, muscle spasms, seizures, nausea, and vomiting.

Trace minerals are required in small amounts in our body. These minute minerals include **iron, zinc, copper, selenium, iodine, chromium, manganese,** and **molybdenum.**

Ultra-trace minerals include **boron, nickel, silicon, arsenic,** and **vanadium** and are necessary for a healthy metabolism.

Water

Though we take it for granted, water is extremely important to our health. Fifty to seventy percent of our body weight (about ten gallons) is water. Since we have no place to store it in our bodies, we cannot live long without it. Water is found inside cells (intracellular) and outside the cells or in the bloodstream (extracellular).

Water is used to regulate body temperatures and helps eliminate waste products through the urine, lungs, skin, and bowels. We need about eight to ten cups a day (one-half ounce per pound of ideal body weight) to maintain this delicate balance.

Our body is a finely tuned machine that requires the right proportions of the nutrients. If one nutrient is out of whack, then others follow and we begin to suffer. It is hard to lose weight when you are out of balance.

Well, nutrition class 101 is now adjourned. Now go eat fit so you can stay fit!

CHAPTER 5

Chronic Inflammation and Antioxidants

"Just push yourself away from the table with your hands and not your belly."
"All you have to do to lose weight is eat less and exercise more."
"It is all a matter of willpower."

Have you heard people make these comments? They reflect our ignorance about the problem of obesity, and why our flawed thinking is accelerating our demise.

You have now arrived at the key chapter in understanding how obesity, metabolic syndrome, type 2 diabetes, high blood pressure, high cholesterol, cancer, and heart disease are all related. This chapter will show you how similar they are, and that by preventing one you might be able to prevent others. *We are not making any claims, just observations.*

How is this for a bold statement? **Obese individuals are starving to death in an overabundance of food.** How can this be?

First of all, you have to realize that obesity is a chronic inflammatory disease and not a character flaw or a matter of willpower (try holding your breath for five minutes to see how much willpower you have). Obese people are sick but think they are healthy.

This chronic inflammation, low-grade inflammation, or "silent inflammation"[30] is a pathway by which diseases like high blood pressure, heart attacks, strokes, type 2 diabetes, some cancers, and obesity affect your body. In addition, inflammation is caused by free-radical damage or can lead to free-radical damage of the tissue and DNA (more about this later).

M. D. Anderson Cancer Center discusses the relationship between inflammation and cancer in a 2010 article:

> This indicates that lifestyle plays a major role in the development of cancer. The important lifestyle factors that affect the incidence and mortality of cancer include tobacco, alcohol, diet, obesity, infectious agents, environmental pollutants, and radiation. All of these risk factors are linked to each other through inflammation.[31]

Obesity even acts like a cancer. The two diseases are very similar. Dr. Barry Sears, author of The Zone Diet, says in his book *Toxic Fat* that we see the following similarities between the various stages of cancer and obesity:

> Normal: Tumor-free (You are lean, and the blood is not inflamed.)
> Stage 1: Benign tumor (You are fat, but the blood is not inflamed.)
> Stage 2: Slowly spreading tumor (You are lean, and the blood is inflamed.)
> Stage 3: Malignant tumor (You are fat, and the blood is inflamed.)[32]

Energy Storage and Use

To understand this process of inflammation and diseases, we need to take a trip down physiology lane. Hang in there, learning a little science isn't as bad for you as a double cheeseburger with fries and a soda at "Burger Doodle."

Our bodies need energy to function, and we get this energy from the calories we eat. The body converts calories into the energy source used by the cells, which is called ATP (adenosine triphosphate). ATP runs the body's engines, or metabolism. ATP equals energy.

Since your cells can only store about ten seconds' worth of ATP, they need a ready supply. This supply is in the form of stored carbohydrates (glycogen stores—remember your G--string?) or fat in fat cells. Fat can make about three times more ATP than carbohydrates and is your "high-octane" fuel.

It is interesting to note that the body has a limited ability to store carbohydrates and even less of an ability to store protein, but *boy*, can it ever store fat, and you know where! So, fat becomes one of the major sources of energy to replenish ATP in the cells. Bottom line, we eat in order to get enough calories to make ATP to run the ship—simple enough. Hope we haven't lost you.

Next comes the problem in your jeans, I mean, your genes. About 75 percent of people are genetically predisposed to trap fat in their fat cells more easily than others. Metabolic syndrome or insulin resistance syndrome is a major culprit in this process. Take your genes and metabolic syndrome together, and you are trapping fat, or energy, while your body is crying for energy to function. Insulin does not allow the fat cells to release fat for energy because insulin is a *storage* enzyme. Your body keeps yelling, *"Release the grease"* but nothing happens.

So, what's a person to do in such a situation? Your body goes into high gear in its panicked state for energy or calories and makes you constantly hungry. You eat to replenish energy, but high insulin levels cause you to store most of your calories, so you eat some more just to survive. You are starving in a sea of plenty. Overeating is not the primary cause of obesity—it is secondary to genes and insulin resistance. It is all part of the "hostile takeover."

According to Dr. Barry Sears, "If you reduce the body's ability to make ATP from incoming calories...you have to either, (1) eat more, (2) slow down physical activity, or (3) start cannibalizing your muscles and organs to get those extra calories."[33]

Cannibalizing is *not* what you want to happen. You are robbing calories from vital organs and muscles just to survive. The term "sarcopenic weight loss" refers to this and is used to describe starvation states like anorexia nervosa. Sarcopenic weight loss means that the person loses weight, but the weight loss is mostly from muscles and organs. Their total body weight goes down, but their body fat percent increases. They are wasting away.

Now you are starting to see that the biological urge to overeat is not controlled by willpower but by starvation or survival and insulin resistance. By now, you might be wondering, what started this whole mess? How could this happen? The answer is right under your nose—your dinner plate.

Toxic Dinner Plates

Did you know that Western surveys of nutrition reveal that 56 percent of our calories come from three sources of food that were *nonexistent* when our genes developed? [53]

- Refined sugars (cane sugar, corn syrup, high-fructose corn syrup, etc.)
- Bleached flour (white bread, pasta, bagels, donuts, etc.)
- Vegetable oils—trans fats and omega-6s (soybean, sunflower, corn, safflower)

From the book *Anticancer* by David Servan-Schreiber, MD, PhD, we learn the alarming news that these three sources of food "*directly* fuel the growth of cancer":

> When we eat sugar or white flour—foods with a high "glycemic index"—blood levels of glucose rise rapidly. The body immediately releases a dose of insulin to enable the glucose to enter cells. The secretion of insulin is accompanied by the release of another molecule, called IGF (insulin-like growth factor), whose role is to stimulate cell growth. In short, sugar nourishes tissues and makes them grow faster. Furthermore, insulin and IGF have another effect in common: They promote the factors of inflammation which…also stimulate cell growth and act, in turn, as fertilizer for tumors.
>
> All the scientific literature points in the same direction: People who want to protect themselves from cancer should seriously reduce their consumption of processed sugar and bleached flour.[34]

In addition, Dr. Barry Sears and Dr. Servan-Schreiber say that we should bring the daily consumption of omega-3 fatty acids (fish oil, flaxseed, linseed) and omega-6 fatty acids (soybean, sunflower, corn, safflower) to a perfectly balanced ratio of 1:1 (eat the same amount of both) instead of the current ratio of 1:15 or 1:40 (way too much omega-6 fatty acids). In addition, omega-9 fats (oleic acid or olive oil) are neutral fats that do not promote inflammation and should be in your diet.

It is interesting to note that the amount of omega-3s in our food depends upon what the cows and chickens we eat have consumed in their food. Omega-3s, besides being found in fish and flaxseed oil, are found in organic products from grass-fed animals or animals with linseed in their feed. If they eat grass, then the milk, meat, and eggs are perfectly balanced in omega-3s and omega-6s.

You might be asking yourself, why is this information about cancer so important in a weight-loss book? According to Dr. Servan-Schreiber, "We finally have an explanation for the simultaneous epidemics of cancer and obesity....Changes in our diets over the last half century point to the culprit: a dietary imbalance in the ratio of essential fatty acids leading to the incredible overconsumption of omega-6s." [35] He goes on to say that the high refined sugar consumption fuels cancer, metabolic syndrome, and obesity. The final common pathway for these diseases is chronic inflammation, the silent killer.

If we accept that cancer growth and obesity are stimulated by dinner plate toxins, then we should start detoxifying what we eat as a way of detoxifying ourselves. Clearly, there is a connection between the cancer rate and the consumption of meat, cold cuts, and milk products. Countries that consume diets high in vegetables and legumes (peas, beans, lentils) have lower cancer rates. Here are two recommendations from Dr. Servan-Schreiber to slow this process:

- Eat sugar and white flour sparingly. Replace them with agave nectar (or other) for sweetening, and multigrain flour for pastas and breads (or sourdough bread made with traditional leaven).
- Avoid all hydrogenated vegetable fats—trans fats (found in croissants and pastries that are not made with butter)—and all animal fats and omega-6s. Olive oil is an excellent vegetable fat that doesn't promote inflammation. Butter (not margarine) and cheeses that are well balanced in omega-3s may not contribute to inflammation either.

As you can see, our diets are very poor and need improvement. Unfortunately, many times people just want a quick fix. *"Just give me a pill."* That wish almost came true, because a few years ago some researchers proposed a "polypill" that would reduce heart disease rates by more than 80 percent. The "polypill" was a combination of six drugs that reduced different heart risk factors. Fortunately, the idea crashed and burned because of concerns about costs and potential adverse effects of taking six medications at a time. [36]

Dr. Oscar H. Franco of Erasmus University Medical Center in Rotterdam, Netherlands, applied the same approach to diet interventions. He concluded that regular consumption of a small number of foods has the potential for reducing heart disease. He called it the "polymeal."[37] He concluded that this combination would reduce heart disease by 76 percent, which is almost as much as the drugs minus the side effects. The meal consisted of:

- Wine (preferably red): 150 ml/day or five ounces
- Fish: four times a week
- Dark chocolate: 100 grams/day (three ounces)
- Fruit and vegetables: 400 grams/day (ADA recommends five to nine servings)
- Garlic: 2.7 gm/day
- Almonds: 68 gm/day (about 2.5 ounces or a little over half a cup)

An interesting finding was that dark chocolate reduced heart-disease risk at the same level as fruits and vegetables because of its high antioxidant properties (more on this later). Only red wine and garlic were slightly higher.

In her book *The O$_2$ Diet*, Keri Glassman, MS, RD, CDN, states that the following are "foods for a slimmer body":[38]

- almonds
- artichokes
- chili peppers
- fatty fish
- flaxseed
- green tea
- lemon water
- lentils
- red grapefruit
- turnips
- yogurt

All of these foods have high antioxidant benefits and overlap with the "polymeal."

There is no substitute for medicine when you are ill and need it, but what are you doing to prevent disease and promote your own personal wellness? The ancient physician Hippocrates said, "Let food be your medicine and medicine be your food." It still applies today—how come we are not listening? Are we just too inflamed?

Inflammation

Let's take a closer look at inflammation to get a better understanding of what is going wrong.

Acute inflammation is your body's defense mechanism that protects you from a foreign substance or injury. The classic signs of acute inflammation are redness, swelling, warmth, and tenderness. Just think how a cut heals. You experience all of these signs as the body begins the healing process. You can also think of a swollen joint from arthritis or a sprain as inflammation. These are all part of acute inflammation—but what is chronic inflammation or "silent inflammation"? According to Dr. Sears:

> Silent inflammation is simply inflammation that falls below the threshold of perceived pain. That's what makes it so dangerous. You don't take any steps to stop it as it smolders for years, if not decades, eventually erupting into what we call chronic disease....If you have high levels of silent inflammation in your body, even if you are not actively sick, it means that you simply cannot be well.[39]

During chronic or silent inflammation, all the inflammatory pathways are at work producing chemicals and attacking would-be enemies. The white blood cell army is very busy destroying and supposedly protecting you. Unfortunately, you are not aware of any of this until the damage gets too overwhelming and some ugly disease raises their heads, like obesity, heart disease, cancer, arthritis, type 2 diabetes, hypertension, or strokes.

To understand how chronic inflammation works requires another trip back to physiology school. Quit groaning, it won't be that bad.

Chronic inflammation is controlled by chemicals in every cell called eicosanoids. Eicosanoids can be either inflammatory ("bad") or non-inflammatory ("good"), depending upon what is needed by the body. Inflammatory "bad" eicosanoids are made from a toxic fat called arachidonic acid (AA), which is made from omega-6 fatty acids (corn, soybean, sunflower, and safflower oil). Non-inflammatory "good" eicosanoids are made essentially from omega-3s fatty acids in fish oil (EPA).

Because of the excess amount of omega-6 oils and refined carbohydrates in our diets, way too much AA is produced. As a protective mechanism, our bodies store the excess AA in—guess where? It is stored in fat cells to protect us. This is fine for a while until we reach the tipping point, and the healthy fat cell gets sick

47

and releases AA. The first sign of your fat cells getting sicker is an increase in insulin levels due to insulin resistance. This process starts the release of inflammatory chemicals (cytokines) from fat cells that travel throughout the body and cause the "hostile takeover." They have great names such as interleukin-6 (IL-6) and tumor necrosis factor (TNF). Think about those guys the next time you eat poorly.

We highly recommend the book *Toxic Fat* by Dr. Barry Sears, in which he calls the AA excess "toxic fat":

> Understanding that our current obesity crisis is really a cancer epidemic is frightening. Excess AA appears first in the adipose tissue [fat cells], which acts as a toxic waste dump to prevent excess silent inflammation from circulating in the blood. The containment of this toxic fat can be breached due to insulin resistance in the adipose tissue. This is caused by a progressive sickening of otherwise healthy fat cells as AA accumulates in these cells. When good fat turns bad, the stored toxic fat (AA) is released into the bloodstream, which sets the molecular stage to begin the inflammatory attack on the rest of the organs. Just like a cancer, you feel no pain until enough accumulated damage occurs to begin causing organ failure.[40]

From this brief account, you can begin to see how our genes and "maladaptive" diets are creating a global epidemic. People are poisoning themselves with every bite of food they take.

Now let's take a moment and look at the powerful weapons used by the "hostile takeover" army of inflammatory cytokines. Those weapons are called free radicals, and chronic inflammation can be caused by free-radical damage or can create free-radical damage.

Free Radicals

What do we mean by free radicals and free-radical damage? Are they hippies leftover from the 1960s or radical groups running around promoting their cause? Obviously they are neither; rather, they are a natural process that occurs in your body that has gotten out of hand. They are a system of "checks and balances" that has gone awry. Don't skip over the technical stuff below just because it is science. You can handle it.

A paradox of nature is that while your body requires oxygen to exist, oxygen can be a highly reactive molecule that can damage the body by producing substances called reactive oxygen species (ROS) or free radicals. For you chemist and science people, a free radical is any atom or molecule that has a single unpaired electron in an outer shell, making it highly reactive.

You might say free radicals are "rogue" molecules that rob electrons from stable molecules that are then "seduced by the dark side"[41] to become free radicals themselves. This is like a pinball effect that wreaks havoc by damaging cells, DNA, and disrupting bodily processes. This is all part of that "hostile takeover."

Free-radical damage is essentially the same as oxidative damage. Oxidation is the process of adding oxygen to a compound. Think of it as rusting. This process, if left unchecked, can cause serious damage to your cells and DNA, increasing the risk of cancer.[42]

The free radicals or ROS produced in cells have strange chemical names like hydrogen peroxide (H_2O_2), hydroxyl radical (OH), superoxide anion (O2-), hypochlorous acid (HOCl), and peroxide radicals (ROO).

Examples of diseases associated with free-radical damage are some forms of cancer, hardening of the arteries (atherosclerosis), high blood pressure (hypertension), high cholesterol, type-2 diabetes, non-alcohol-induced liver damage, lung disease from cigarette smoking, Parkinson's disease, some forms of deafness, schizophrenia, Alzheimer's, iron storage disease (hemochromatosis), obesity, and the aging process itself. (Other than these diseases, free radicals aren't too serious.)

Diet-Driven Inflammation AGEs You

Silent inflammation can be stimulated at *any age* by diet and cooking at too high temperatures. Did you know that cooking foods at high temperatures (deep frying) results in a "browning" effect, where sugars and certain oxidized fats react with proteins to form a very tissue-damaging protein-sugar compound called advanced glycation end products or AGEs for short? AGEs (and age) accelerate the production of free radicals.

You might say that the normal aging process resembles a slow cooking process. As we "cook," or age, a low-grade, chronic state of inflammation is being created. This process damages our skin, arteries, eye lenses, and cartilage. This all happens by these AGE products "cross-linking" with proteins in our body and making them barely functional. As these damaged proteins begin to accumulate, they accelerate the formation of damaging free radicals—about fifty times the rate of normal proteins. In addition, if that wasn't bad enough, they produce pro-inflammatory messenger chemicals called cytokines, which accelerate the chronic inflammation process.[43]

Think of the AGE proteins looking like an old rubber band that is crusted and has lost its elasticity. It breaks easily, and whatever it is holding gets spilled all over the place. Guess where that is happening—in your body! I love this quote from Kobi Yamada:

If you don't take care of your body, where do you plan to live?

Antioxidants to the Rescue

Antioxidants, on the other hand, are reducing agents that limit oxidative damage by neutralizing free radicals.

Fortunately, Mother Nature (or perhaps a higher power) created a fix for the free-radical problem. "Mother" does know best. She called in her "Auntie O" (Anti Oxidant) to the rescue. Antioxidants disable free radicals by donating electrons to that outer shell to replace those lost during oxidation, thus protecting us.

Remember, not all free-radical damage is bad. The body uses free radicals for protection and garbage removal. For instance, the body uses free radicals to destroy unwanted bacteria, viruses, and cancer cells. Free radicals are a ready-made arsenal of weapons used by your immune system army to destroy unwanted invaders, but they must be kept in check. It's like keeping the arms race in check.

Free radicals are necessary for life, and the body has a number of mechanisms in place to minimize excessive free-radical damage. The function of the antioxidant systems is not to remove these free radicals entirely, but instead to keep them at an optimum level. Again, this is a system of checks and balances.

Names of the antioxidants include superoxide dismutase, catalase, glutathione peroxidase, and glutathione reductase. In addition, when you are under attack by free radicals, you need some "ACEs" up your sleeve—vitamin A, vitamin C, vitamin E, and selenium. Further, there is good evidence that bilirubin and uric acid can act as antioxidants.[44]

The colors in plants (called polyphenols and carotenoids) come from pigments that protect the seeds from the direct rays of the sun and are very beneficial to us. These colors are the antioxidants. You are probably familiar with the red and purple colors of berries, the orange of an orange, yellow of a lemon, and the red of a tomato. All of these plant pigments make up the protective antioxidants that we need. Another subclass of antioxidants is the colorless flavanols found in cocoa.[45]

Antioxidants are found in varying amounts in foods such as fruits and vegetables like apples, onions, soybeans, blueberries, pomegranate, cranberries, and acai berry. In addition, antioxidants can be found in other foods like red wine, dark chocolate, teas (green and black), whole grains (not processed flour), legumes (beans, peas), spices, and nuts. Note that processed foods contain fewer antioxidants than fresh or uncooked foods because the processing destroys the antioxidants.

Therefore, the more fresh, whole foods we eat, the more we reduce inflammation and the likelihood of inflammation-related diseases:

> Much evidence indicates that certain constituents of fruits, vegetables, nuts, legumes, and spices can down regulate inflammation [prevent or improve] and most chronic diseases. Flavonoids are one category of nutraceuticals present in these dietary products that can suppress inflammation and thus play an important role in inflammation-related diseases, including cancer.
> The health benefits of wine, chocolates, fruits, vegetables, nuts, spices, and legumes are attributable to their flavonoids [antioxidants].[46]

It must be noted that people who consume diets high in fruits and vegetables have lower risk of certain cancers, heart disease, and diabetes according to the National Cancer Institute—but this protection does *not* hold true for white potatoes. The skin of white potatoes does have some antioxidant value, but the starchy white part does not.

According to the NHANES II study, do you know what is the number-one vegetable eaten by Americans? Guess! You'll find the answer after the next section.

Anti-inflammatory and Antioxidant Foods

It isn't possible to overstate how important diet is in relation to your health: [48]

The highly processed, calorie-dense, nutrient-depleted diet favored in the current American culture frequently leads to exaggerated...post-prandial [after eating] spikes in blood glucose and lipids [fats]. This state...induces immediate oxidant stress, which increases in direct proportion to the increases in glucose and triglycerides [fats] after a meal. The transient increase in free radicals acutely triggers atherogenic changes [hardening of the arteries] including inflammation, endothelial dysfunction [lining of arteries disrupted], hypercoagulability [increased blood clotting], and sympathetic hyperactivity...increased risk of future cardiovascular events [heart attacks] even in nondiabetic individuals.

Improvements in diet exert profound and immediate favorable changes in these...disturbances. Low glycemic index vegetables and fruits, nuts, lean protein, vinegar, tea, fish oil, calorie restriction, weight loss, and moderate- to low-dose alcohol each significantly improve post-meal inflammation. This anti-inflammatory diet should be considered for the primary and secondary prevention of coronary artery disease and diabetes.[47]

This article goes on to say that chronic inflammation is increasingly recognized as a cause of heart disease, diabetes, and Alzheimer disease, and that a "maladaptive diet" is a major underlying cause of this chronic inflammation. This occurs when too many refined carbohydrates (sugar, starch, white flour, etc.) and the wrong type of fats (omega-6, trans fats, and saturated fats) are eaten during a meal. This type of a meal generates excess free radicals (or reactive oxygen species) that stimulate a cascade resulting in inflammation and eventually heart problems (coronary artery disease).

Recent studies indicated that about one-third of Americans and two-thirds of heart patients have abnormal blood sugars—prediabetic or diabetic—because of their diets. That is alarming! In addition, a *single meal* high in saturated fat will shower the bloodstream with fats, oxidative stress, and inflammation. This is independent of the highly refined carbohydrate diet. The two together are even worse. These findings are common manifestations of the metabolic syndrome, which is a prediabetic state.

This excessive eating of refined carbohydrates and the wrong kind of fats causes surges in blood sugar and fat levels (triglycerides). This surge overwhelms the body and leads to the creation of free radicals, which fuels the fire of inflammation.[48]

In addition to free-radical damage, sugar can cause another very annoying problem. It has been found that fructose-rich beverages like sugar-sweetened sodas and fruit juices are associated with an increased risk of developing gout in men and women. Gouty arthritis is very painful, and gout can lead to the painful condition of uric acid kidney stones.[49]

Are you beginning to feel that our dinner plates are becoming our worst enemy?

Antioxidant supplementations have the potential to alleviate the hardening of the arteries caused by excessive production of reactive oxygen species (free radicals). A recent study published in 2010 stated that "Antioxidant supplementation significantly increased large and small artery elasticity in patients with multiple cardiovascular [heart] risk factors. This beneficial vascular effect was associated with an improvement in glucose and lipid metabolism as well as decrease in blood pressure."[50]

As you can now see, obesity, cancer, heart disease, type 2 diabetes, high cholesterol, and high blood pressure are all related and interact through chronic inflammation.

Proper diet and high-antioxidant foods should play a major part in your overall health and well-being. Heart disease, which is still the number-one killer of both men and women, is the end result of inflammation and free-radical damage caused by metabolic syndrome, diabetes, high lipids, and obesity. Therefore it is majorly important to tailor your diet, exercise, and lifestyle in a much healthier direction. Antioxidants are a major step along the way, but how do we know what to look for and which foods are better?

Answer to question: The number-one consumed vegetable in America is French fries (25 percent of all vegetables eaten). Next comes ketchup, pizza sauce, and onions.[51] *Now how is that for a formula for disease?* **It's job security for physicians.**

More Very Important Science "Stuff"

Before moving onto antioxidant and anti-inflammatory foods, let's take a minute and talk about real science "stuff." You may soon come across these very technical compounds, and you need to be aware of them. They are the cutting edge of research on inflammation and its relationship to obesity, diabetes, heart disease, and some cancers.

The first substance is nuclear factor-kappa beta (NF-kB). *Don't gag on the name, just pay attention, this is important.* NF-kB is a protein complex that controls the transcription of DNA in most cells of the body. A transcription factor simply turns on your DNA (genes), allowing it to send its message to the body. *NF-kB is the rapid response team that turns on inflammation when your body needs it* and is activated by stress, cytokines, free radicals, ultraviolet irradiation, oxidized LDL, bacteria, and viruses.

NF-kB is beneficial for the protection of the body, but when you consume a poor diet high in refined carbohydrates, too many omega-6 fats (corn, safflower, and soybean), and not enough omega-3 fish oils, NF-kB becomes one of the chief culprits in chronic inflammation, causing the immune system not to work properly and resulting in the development of diseases like metabolic syndrome, diabetes, heart disease, and cancer.[52]

Controlling NF-kB helps control chronic inflammation, and that starts with a proper diet. Many natural-food products include antioxidants that have anti-inflammatory activity and inhibit NF-kB. Appendix D contains an anti-inflammatory food pyramid.

Next is the sirtuin I protein, or SIRT I, which is known as the "skinny gene." This protein increases insulin sensitivity and counters metabolic syndrome. Anti-inflammatory foods that turn SIRT I on help protect you from the destruction of chronic inflammation. Again, it all starts with your diet.

Let's move onto examining these wonderfully protective foods.

Measuring Antioxidant Levels in Foods

So, just how powerful is one antioxidant-containing food compared to another? That is hard to say because almost every manufacturer of health foods makes a more outlandish claim than their competitor. **In addition, not all antioxidants are anti-inflammatory.** How do we know?

Welcome the new sheriff to town. His name is Officer ORAC.

ORAC is an acronym for oxygen radical absorbance capacity. It is an analysis that measures the total antioxidant power of foods in a test tube (in vitro). The Total ORAC 5.0™ tests the antioxidant protection against five major free radicals found in the human body. They are peroxynitrite, super oxide anion, peroxyl radicals, hydroxyl radicals, and single oxygen.

Chronic Inflammation and Antioxidants

In a study done in 1999 at the Human Nutrition Research Center on Aging at Tufts in Boston, eating plenty of high-ORAC foods "raised the antioxidant power of human blood 10% to 25%."[53] Here is a list of the top-scoring ORAC fruits and vegetables.

Top-Scoring Fruits and Vegetables
USDA Data on Foods with High ORAC Scores

Food	Serving Size	Antioxidant Capacity Per Serving Size
Raw unprocessed cocoa	100 grams	28000
Small red bean	½ cup dried	13727
Wild blueberry	1 cup	13427
Red kidney bean	½ cup dried	13259
Pinto bean	½ cup	11864
Blueberry	1 cup (cultivated)	9019
Cranberry	1 cup (whole)	8983
Artichoke hearts	1 cup (cooked)	7904
Blackberry	1 cup (cultivated)	7701
Prune	½ cup	7291
Raspberry	1 cup	6058
Strawberry	1 cup	5938
Red Delicious apple	1 apple	5900
Granny Smith apple	1 apple	5381
Pecan	1 ounce	5095
Sweet cherry	1 cup	4873
Black plum	1 plum	4844
Russet potato	1 (cooked)	4649
Black bean	½ cup dried	4181
Plum	1 plum	4118
Gala apple	1 apple	3903

One extremely good antioxidant food is not on this list. You will never guess. The super food is beets. The red pigment is a very high source of antioxidants that help protect against cancer and obesity.

Without looking back on the chart, rate the following foods from the highest antioxidant value to the lowest: blueberries, pecans, small red beans, and a Red Delicious apple. What is your answer?

In order of highest antioxidant value: small red beans, blueberries, Red Delicious apple, and pecans. The point of the quiz is to think of other foods besides fruit as being high in antioxidants. You need a variety.

Please be aware that with nearly all vegetables, conventional boiling can reduce the ORAC value by up to 90 percent, while steaming retains more of the antioxidants.

The amount of a food also determines how high its ORAC score is; for example, one cup of sweet cherries has about the same ORAC as one black plum. Make sure you are comparing "apples to apples" in terms of serving size; otherwise the ORAC scores of one food might look falsely higher or lower in comparison to a similar food.[54]

Healthy Chocolate?

Over the last several years, scientists have discovered that one food, long thought of as "junk food," can actually contribute to healthy and lasting weight loss. So what food is it?

Chocolate! That's right, chocolate.

Of course, not just any chocolate will do the trick (in fact, the more common forms of "candy" chocolate are contributors to the obesity epidemic). But findings from numerous studies show that dark chocolate that is cold processed, high in natural cocoa ingredients, and devoid of processed sugars, hydrogenated oils, and other artificial ingredients can provide the body with a powerful antioxidant weight-control tool.

According to a study published in 2005, "Dark chocolate improves insulin sensitivity and resistance and decreases blood pressure, whereas white chocolate does not....Numerous studies indicate that flavanols may exert significant vascular protection because of their antioxidant properties."[55]

In the book *The Healing Powers of Chocolate*, Keri Gans, RD, is quoted as stating, "Dark chocolate on a per-weight basis has the highest concentration of flavonoids of any food. Dark chocolate is loaded with a variety of phytonutrients, making it extremely high in antioxidants."[56] You might just say that it is a **healthy chocolate.**

The following table shows the antioxidant (flavanol) content of three different types of chocolate. As you can see, dark chocolate (70 percent cocoa) is far superior.[57]

Type of Chocolate	Phenolics (mg/100g)	Flavonoids (mg/100g)
Dark chocolate	57,867	2830
Milk chocolate	16,046	1,348
White chocolate	12,639	770

Here are some thoughts on chocolate from Cleone Lyvonne, the author of *Abracadabra: I Weigh What I Want to Weigh*:

> When I eat chocolate, I really LIVE IN THE MOMENT, concentrate on every bite, and enjoy it to the nth degree. Why eat it if you aren't going to ENJOY it!!!??? When people eat it fast, and/or while doing something else, and don't concentrate, they deprive themselves of pleasure and often end up feeling not only dissatisfied but also guilty! What a waste of calories.[58]

Besides being pleasurable, the health benefits of dark chocolate are numerous. They range from weight loss to cardiovascular benefits to mood altering to dental health and many more

Dark chocolate benefits the heart and circulatory system through its anti-inflammatory effect. This effect helps prevent oxidation of LDL cholesterol (remember, L = Lousy, and oxidation of LDL cholesterol causes hardening of the arteries) and reduces platelet stickiness (aka sludge—not good). According to a 2004 article published in *U.S. Pharmacist*, "dietary chocolate...can be used as a functional food to help reduce coronary heart disease risk for people with mild hypercholesterolemia [high cholesterol]."[59] In addition, "eating dark chocolate would afford the same protection against cardiovascular diseases [heart disease] as green tea."[60]

According to a study published in 2005, eating cocoa can help reduce high-fat, diet-induced obesity by altering fat metabolism, especially by decreasing fatty-acid production. In this study the cocoa worked by regulating the genes for fat production.[61]

In addition, dark chocolate can lower blood pressure, help lower blood sugar, improve insulin sensitivity/resistance, help diabetes, improve blood vessels (protective vascular endothelium), "thin the blood" (decrease platelet adhesiveness or stickiness), help fight depression, and promote dental health.[62] And consider this: by simply smelling dark chocolate, you can decrease your appetite and reduce levels of ghrelin, a hormone secreted by the stomach that increases appetite.[63] How is that for chocolate being a powerful stimulant?

As research continues, more and more beneficial uses of chocolate are being discovered.

You might say, "A chocolate a day keeps the doctor away."

The "Spice of Life"

Chocolate is not the only delicious food source of antioxidant and anti-inflammatory properties:

> Extensive research within the past two decades has revealed that obesity is an inflammatory disease. Several spices have been shown to exhibit activity against obesity through antioxidant and anti-inflammatory mechanisms. Among them, curcumin, a yellow pigment derived from the spice turmeric (an essential component of curry powder), has been investigated most extensively as a treatment for obesity and obesity-related metabolic diseases. These curcumin-induced alterations reverse insulin resistance, hyperglycemia [high blood sugar], hyperlipidemia [high cholesterol], and other symptoms linked to obesity. Other structurally homologous nutraceuticals, derived from red chili, cinnamon, cloves, black pepper, and ginger, also exhibit effects against obesity and insulin resistance.[64]

There are over three hundred reports published on curcumin, a natural antioxidant, and its effects on obesity and obesity-associated complications. "Several reports suggest that curcumin has potential in the prevention and treatment of obesity, diabetes, atherosclerosis, and metabolic syndrome."[65] Basically, curcumin counterattacks the "hostile takeover." Some researchers believe that it is the most powerful antioxidant and anti-inflammatory product available naturally. For better absorption of curcumin, it should be taken with the pepper extract bioperidine.

In addition to curcumin, there are many reports that other spice nutraceuticals may also affect obesity and insulin resistance by attacking the inflammatory pathways. The other powerful spices include capsaicin from red chili, piperine from black pepper, eugenol from cloves, and gingerol from ginger. In addition, garlic, onions, red pepper, fenugreek, and cinnamon have also been shown to have beneficial effects.

Special note should be given to another naturally occurring substance called Boswellia serrata, which is a form of Indian frankincense. Studies have shown it to have very strong antioxidant and anti-inflammatory properties. It assists in neutralizing immunopathological disorders causing chronic inflammation like Crohn's disease, ulcerative colitis, rheumatoid arthritis, and osteoarthritis.[66]

Because of the low cost of these spices, their safety, and the evidence of their effectiveness, it is essential to include them as a part of your daily diet. They definitely are your "spice of life."

As you can see, antioxidant and anti-inflammatory foods are essential components in the battle against obesity and many other related diseases. **Fruits, vegetables, and spices are God's vitamin pills to us, and we should consume them in abundance.** At least get your five to nine servings a day (ten to fifteen servings are better, and the more colors the better), every day, and make sure you spice up your life.

But—

"Houston, we have a problem."

These are the words from *Apollo 13* on its space mission when a major problem occurred. Unfortunately, the problem for us is that **people two years and older on average consume only 2.6 servings of fruits and vegetables per day.** To make things worse, about one-third of those servings were starches like white potatoes.[67] Where are people going to get vitamins, minerals, or phytonutrients for good health if they are not eating fruits and vegetables? **THEY AREN'T!** This definitely is a formula for disease and suffering.

Fortunately we've provided Appendices C and D, which include a listing of anti-inflammatory foods.

Carotenoids and Algae

The natural world around us abounds with color from leaves, flowers, fruits, vegetables, and animals. Everywhere we look we are greeted with an abundance of vivid colors spanning the spectrum of the rainbow. According to Kazunaga Yazawa, PhD, professor of Nutraceuticals and Functional Foods at Tokyo University of Marine Science and Technology, "These colors, acquired historically by flora and fauna from experience as 'living wisdom,' are a major blessing for humans as well. For research in recent years has demonstrated that locked away secretly in natural colors lay unmatched power for human health."[68] One of the most representative groups of natural colors are carotenoids, which are pigments that account for 0.1 percent of the natural organic compounds found on Earth. Each year plants produce forty million tons of carotenoids, and as of 2005 over seven hundred different kinds have been identified.[69]

You can find carotenoids in a wide range of foods. They include beta-carotene from carrots, lycopene from tomatoes, lutein from egg yolks, capsanthin from paprika, and astaxanthin from salmon flesh and the shells of shrimp and crabs. The reason carotenoids are so important is they are strong antioxidants that fight free radicals.

One carotenoid of interest is astaxanthin, which causes the red color in shrimp, crab, and salmon. It has been shown to improve eye fatigue, reduce high blood pressure (hypertension), help maintain skin health while reducing wrinkles, help reduce type 2 diabetes, improve weight loss, and improve physical endurance and muscle recovery—all of this in a little red pigment from the sea.[70]

Become Radically Free

So, what is the secret of being "radically free" in your diet?

- Cut out the refined carbohydrates (white bread, bagels, donuts, white rice, white potatoes, white flour).
- Minimize consumption of omega-6s fats (corn, soybean, sunflower, and safflower).
- Increase your consumption of omega-3s (fish oil, flaxseed).
- Eat omega-9s (olive, canola).
- Eat dark chocolate.
- Eat a variety of spices (curcumin, cinnamon, ginger, pepper).
- Eat dark chocolate.
- Consume more green vegetables.

- Eat more dark chocolate.
- Eat beets.
- Eat more dark chocolate.
- Consume lower-glycemic-level fruit (blueberries, cherries)
- Eat more dark chocolate.
- Drink some red wine (one glass for women and two for men).
- Eat more dark chocolate.

This is the secret of becoming "radically free" of free radicals and inflammation. It is right under your nose three times a day.

CHAPTER 6

Exercise

Exercise (ek'ser'siz'), n: The ancient art of converting large meals and wonderfully fattening food into pulled muscles and back strains by lifting extremely heavy objects that don't need lifting and running when no one is chasing you.

(Unknown author)

Unfortunately, it's pretty clear that definition above is probably most people's opinion of exercise. It seems like this trend of inactivity has been going on for a while and is getting worse. According to the American College of Sports Medicine (ACSM), "More than 60% of American adults are not regularly physically active. In fact, 25% of all adults are not active at all."[71]

Well, so much for the exercise craze that is sweeping the nation. Actually, it's probably a couch-potato craze that is sweeping the nation. So how do we deal with this phenomenon?

We return to school and start Couch Potato Workout 101. Does that mean that you run a marathon on your first day? Absolutely not! (Just on the second day—just kidding!) Overdoing an exercise program gets you sore, discouraged, and ready to quit before you even begin. **So, start slowly if you are not used to exercising.**

Activity Verses Exercise

You may have wondered about the difference between activity and exercise. Whether or not that question has ever crossed your mind, we are going to tell you. According to the US Department of Health and Human Services, these are the definitions:

Physical activity is any bodily movement produced by skeletal muscle resulting in energy expenditure. Examples are walking, running, household chores, playing sports, etc.

Exercise is physical activity that is planned or structured. It involves repetitive bodily movement aimed to improve physical fitness (cardio, flexibility, muscle strength training).

As you can see, exercise is a category of physical activity. In addition, there is a very NEAT category also under physical activity.

A Very NEAT Activity

NEAT stands for non-exercise activity thermogenesis. Now, before you go, "Oh brother, what did he just say?" let me translate. Non-exercise means it is not planned, just like our definition above says. It is an occupational activity, a leisure-time activity, like running errands, shopping, yard work, or household activity. Thermogenesis simply means burning of calories or creating heat.

Many times when we go to the gym and exercise, we think that is enough. It's possible to assume that you can become a couch potato for the rest of the day since you already exercised. Don't fall into that trap. Since activity accounts for about 20 percent of your daily calories burned, keeping active is important. Don't just rely on your workout, if you even did one.

A study done of thirteen thousand men over seven years showed that leisure-time activity (bowling, fishing, light walking, yard work, etc.) lowered the risk of heart disease by 20 percent.[72] *So, get moving.*

You may have heard that exercise is more important in the maintenance phase than the weight-loss phase. This is true, but why? Be aware that we are not saying exercise is not important for weight loss; we are saying that it is more important in maintenance.

Let's say you lost forty pounds. You are a now a lighter person moving around, and it takes less energy to do your daily activities. Wouldn't you agree that if I strapped on a forty-pound weight to you and had you carry it around all day that you would burn a lot more energy? The reverse is true if you lose the weight. You burn less. Therefore, exercising an hour a day and burning four hundred calories like the participants in the National Weight Control Registry (more about them later) will help you burn the calories that you are no longer burning up carrying the extra forty pounds.

The best way to begin exercising is to walk. The best way to accomplish this walking goal is to purchase a pedometer and measure how many steps you take a day. Any sporting-goods store or major chain will have pedometers. The average person walks three thousand to four thousand steps per day. Your goal is to do a 10K every day. That is, ten thousand steps per day. For every two thousand steps you walk (that is approximately one mile), you burn about one hundred calories.

Measure your average distance for the first week. Try to increase your distance by 50 percent every one to two weeks. For example, if you walk three thousand steps per day this week, try to increase your distance to four thousand five hundred steps per day next week. When you feel comfortable with that distance, increase it another 50 percent. By increasing to ten thousand steps per day you will be walking five miles and burning approximately five hundred calories per day.

Walking can be done outside, in a mall, in a gym, on a treadmill in your home, or throughout the office or place where you work. Add extra steps by parking farther from the store, office, or shop. Take the stairs when you can. They all count. Whether you walk or run the steps, calories you burn will be about the same. Running is just faster, as well as offering some aerobic benefit.

Studies have shown that you do not have to do your walking all at once.[73] You can do increments of ten to fifteen minutes throughout the day. They all count for the total of your steps. Walking at a moderate pace for ten-minute intervals throughout the day (on a lunch break, walking the dog, before and after work, or doing errands) counts. Just do it because it is not that hard. If you want, make it into a fun game. Say to yourself, "OK, pedometer, I'm going to beat you today. You are not going to get the best of me, you little sucker."

Once you become more advanced in your workouts, you may want to follow the ACSM guidelines for aerobic activity. Aerobic activity, endurance training, or "cardio" is low-intensity exercise that raises your heart rate and keeps it elevated for a period of time, which is usually greater than seven minutes. You might want to consult a certified trainer familiar with these guidelines. Good certifications to look for are ACSM, ACE, or CHEK.

The guidelines for aerobic activity include:

1. Exercise: At least five days per week at moderate intensity or three days a week at vigorous intensity.
2. Warm up: five to ten minutes at low intensity before aerobic activity.
3. Conditioning: twenty to sixty minutes of aerobic or resistance activity.
4. Cool down: five to ten minutes at low intensity.
5. Stretching: ten minutes after the warm-up or cool-down phase. The stretch should be held for fifteen to sixty seconds.[74]

The intensity of your exercise can be measured by target heart rate. The standard way of calculating target heart rate is to subtract your age from 220. That gives an estimation of your maximum heart rate. The ACSM recommends that you exercise at 65 to 80 percent of your maximum heart rate.

For example, if you are fifty years old, 220 – 50 = 170, or your maximum heart rate. Taking 65 percent of 170 is a 110 heart rate (0.65 x 170 = 110) and taking 80 percent of 170 is a 136 (0.8 x 170 = 136) heart rate. Therefore, a fifty-year-old should exercise at a heart rate of 110 to 136 beats per minute to achieve an aerobic workout.

As always, consult your physician before starting any exercise program.

Don't forget strength training. This includes weight lifting or anaerobic exercise and provides a number of very important benefits. Strength training helps build muscle and build and strengthen bones, improves quality of life, and promotes independent living. One of the best predictors of how well you will survive an illness, surgery, or injury after age sixty-five is muscle mass, which is protein. The more muscle you have, the better chance you have of recovering.

The increased muscle mass also increases your metabolism and burns calories. Muscle burns many more calories than fat does.

Strength training can be done on the same or a separate day as endurance or aerobic training. It is a higher intensity but lower duration exercise. Lifting weights can be done with machines, bands, or free weights, and this type of training only needs to be done two to three times per week, along with your cardiovascular training, to achieve improvement in your physical fitness.[75]

You might be asking yourself, "Do I need to do both types of exercise—cardio and strength training?" An article published in *JAMA* in 2010 studied this question in diabetics, which could apply to everyone. They found that only the combination of resistance and cardio (aerobic) training was associated with improvements in blood sugar control.[76] The bottom line is you should do both types of exercise. *Quit groaning!*

Don't forget that when you are strength training to gain muscle, you need to consume more complete high-quality protein in your diet. The American Dietetic Association recommends 0.8 grams of protein for every kilogram you weigh (0.4 grams per pound), but if your are intensely training, men need 1.5 grams per kilogram (0.7 grams per pound) and women need 1.2 grams per kilogram (0.5 grams per pound). (Sorry for the complicated math.) For example, a female athlete weighing 140 pounds, would multiply her weight of 140 pounds by 0.5 grams per pound (140 x 0.5 = 70). She needs seventy grams a day of protein to maintain working out as an athlete. For everyone else, just multiply your weight by 0.4 for your daily grams of protein needed (140 x 0.4 = 56 grams). Also, when in doubt, eat more protein. But remember, cooked meat, fish, or fowl has seven grams of protein per ounce, so you only need four to five ounces per serving three or four times a day.

Once you become more advanced in your workouts, you may want to use a certified personal trainer. Again, make sure he or she is certified by a nationally recognized organization mentioned above.

Have you heard the expression "putty in my hands"? Well, if you decide not to exercise, you will become a big blob of putty in your caregiver's hands. That is not where you want to be. So, the bottom line is, move it or lose it! The choice is yours. No more excuses!

CHAPTER 7

The Environment

Have we gotten to the point that we have to put a skull and crossbones on our food labels and menus? It might not be such a bad idea. Just read these quotes:

> People with weight problems face a difficult, even toxic environment. The temptations to eat are constant, powerful, and compelling. If you pause for a moment to think, you might be surprised by how we accept this without the slightest protest.[77]

Here is an interesting statement from Brian Wansink, PhD, professor of marketing and nutrition science and director of the Food Brand Laboratory, University of Illinois:

Personally, I believe it's just too difficult for the average person to constantly remind themselves to not eat those cookies, to skip the fries, or to pass on the extra handful of M&Ms. Because of this, I believe we'd be better off trying to change or control our environment in a way that helps make better, healthier food choices. Better yet, create an environment that eliminates poor nutrition choices as salient options.[78]

Now let's factor in a statement about our genetics from George Bray, MD, renowned obesity expert from Louisiana State University: "Genetics is the loaded gun, but environment is the trigger that fires the gun."

Putting it all together, we discover that our "toxic environment" and poor food choices can trigger a person who is genetically predisposed to become obese or overweight.

It is interesting to note that our stomachs don't come with a fuel gauge that tells us when enough fuel has been consumed. You might think that fullness or satiety is enough, but consider this. It takes the brain about twenty minutes to let you know that you are full. Most people eat their food in ten minutes, so they have a tendency to overeat because they have not yet experienced fullness. Overeating an extra hundred calories a day (two medium cookies) can add ten pounds of weight in one year. Since the average weight gain for Americans is about 1 to 3 percent per year, there seems to be a lot of broken fuel gauges.[79]

Also, as you start eating something, the evidence disappears and "food amnesia" takes over. This all clouds your thinking as to how much you should be eating and how much you have eaten. Normal-weight people **underestimate** their calories by 10 to 20 percent and overweight people underestimate their calories by 30 to 40 percent.[80]

It is very important to focus on factors in your environment that cause you to unknowingly overeat. Many of these "hidden persuaders" affect you on an unconscious level and can indeed be very powerful.

Hidden Persuaders in a "Toxic Environment"

There are four environmental factors that play into American's expanding waistline. They are packaging, convenience, variety, and cost.[81]

The Environment

Packaging

Your overconsumption of a product can be greatly influenced by packaging. Dr. Wansink discusses an interesting study on how much food people ate based on the size of a package it came in:

> In a recent study, we gave half of our participant's half-pound bags of M&Ms and the other half two-pound bags, each group with instructions to watch an accompanying video. At the end of the video we measured how many M&Ms were eaten, and we found those people with two-pound bags ate more than twice the amount of M&Ms than those people with the half-pound bags ate.[82]

From this and other studies we learn that larger package sizes encourage people to consume 19 to 45 percent more food. It is better to buy individual serving sizes instead of the large economy size. The economic savings will be in your waistline.

Convenience

Anytime you have an urge to eat, you can satisfy that urge quickly and conveniently. Almost anywhere you can find soda and junk-food vending machines, and almost every corner has a fast-food restaurant.

Processed foods that are "good tasting" and easy to make are included in the convenience category. Grocery stores carry the microwave, frozen, quickie meals that are ready to go. "Nuke" it and you're ready. It almost makes you wonder why we have kitchens any more.

Variety

A variety of convenience foods comes next. We have for your liking "Burger Doodle," "Taco Doodle," "Southern Fried Chicken Doodle," and "Pizza Doodle." If you are one of the many people who eat fast food several times a week, you are in variety heaven. When you tire of one, there is always another. *I guess we need to quit doodling.*

Have you ever wondered how the fast-food restaurants can keep you coming back? Well, many of the tastes and aromas of these "luscious" foods are manufactured at a series of large chemical plants by flavor chemists:

> About 90 percent of the money that Americans spend on food is used to buy processed food. But the canning, freezing, and dehydrating techniques used to process food destroy most of its flavor. Since the end of

World War II, a vast industry has arisen in the United States to make processed food palatable. Without this flavor industry, today's fast-food industry could not exist. The names of the leading American fast-food chains and their best-selling menu items have become famous world-wide, embedded in our popular culture. Few people, however, can name the companies that manufacture fast food's taste. The flavor industry is highly secretive.[83]

So, go enjoy an ethyl-2-methyl-butyrate covered with ethyl-3-hydroxybutanoate. Add a serving of methyl-2 paraldehyde-ketone and enjoy. Those are the flavors of an apple with marshmallow along with a serving of popcorn. Enjoy the aroma of PJR3X6660032 being pumped through the ventilation system that smells like grilled burgers and fries.

Bon appétit!

Cost

The amount of food or calories you get at fast-food restaurants is cheap for the price. That is, if you deduct medical costs, higher medical-insurance premiums, and doctor's fees:

> In 1970, Americans spent about $6 billion on fast food; in 2001 they spent more than $110 billion. Americans now spend more money on fast food than on higher education, personal computer, computer soft-ware, or new cars. They spend more on fast food than on movies, books, magazines, newspapers, videos, and recorded music—combined.[84]

The combination of packaging, convenience, variety, and cost are definitely fueling our addiction to fast foods. Then we wonder why our country is having trouble with its waistline.

Grocery Shopping

Grocery shopping can offer some unique challenges also. The arrangement of products is scientifically designed. For instance, notice on what shelf they put sugar cereals—eye level for little kids. If you think only children are affected by placement, consider that there is a 40 percent increase in sales of items placed on the end of aisles even if the item isn't on sale. People will purchase up to 30 percent more when they are exposed to multiple-unit pricing (e.g., 3 for $3 versus 1 for $1).[85]

To help with grocery-store shopping, Dr. Wansink suggests grocery lists are not always good because they often increase the time you spend in the store, which increases the chances of impulse buying. He suggests that you give yourself a time limit. Even write it on the top of the grocery list. He also mentions that people "zigzag" shop through the store up and down each aisle, which causes them to purchase more than they intended to purchase.

Instead, he suggests "spot shopping," which is mission-focused. You write down the four or five items that you need and where you think they are located in the store. *Your mission, should you choose to accept it,* is to get your items and GET OUT. It is interesting that his studies have shown that 93 percent of all people surveyed have an unused item in their cupboard that is over three years old.

Also keep in mind that even though an item may be somewhat more expensive if purchased in smaller, individual serving sizes, it might be the most economical from an over-consumption perspective.

Start by going through your cupboards and refrigerator and throwing away all bad choices of food. If it's not there, you will not be tempted to eat it. Literally, this is "out of sight, out of mind."

We know that you don't want to let any food go to waste by throwing it out, but you can spell waste two ways, so which *waist/waste* are you talking about? Why not donate it to a local food bank?

CHAPTER 8

The "Nuts and Bolts" of How to Do It

If you only read one chapter in this book, this should be it. It is the nuts and bolts of a successful weight-loss program. The steps will seem simple and easy, but remember there is a huge amount of science behind them. The whole concept can be summarized in this very "technical" statement, which is a popular English nursery rhyme from 1806.

Twinkle, twinkle, little star
How I wonder what you are!
Up above the world so high
Like a diamond in the sky!

So, what does a nursery rhyme have to do with a weight-loss program? First, you can go outside on a beautiful clear night and enjoy the twinkle of the little stars; so simple and so easy to enjoy. There is nothing to it, but what are stars? Stars are raging infernos of burning gas, planets, galaxies, novas, supernovas, black holes, trillions of them, millions of miles away, and some are much larger than our sun. They are anything but simple. They are quite enormous and complex, yet they are "like a diamond in the sky."

So it is with this weight-loss program. It will look very simple, like the stars, but it is backed with supernova-like science and raging infernos of published studies. This book can help you understand some of the science, but all you really need to know is:

"This is how we do it."

Now, let's go onto the nuts and bolts of the program. Just eat nuts and bolts and you won't have room for food. Besides, you will be extremely full for a long time.

Weight-Loss Program

Before beginning, let's distinguish between weight loss and weight maintenance. They are two distinctly different areas in managing your weight. The weight-loss phase usually lasts one to six months. That is the active phase, and calorie restriction is common.

Maintenance is hanging onto what you lose—keeping the weight off. Chapter 9 is devoted to maintenance, and **maintenance should last for two years after you reach your goal weight. If you are a diabetic, it should last for four years after you reach your goal weight.**[86]

Notice that surgery and medications will not be discussed. Sometimes these treatments are necessary, but you need to be under the care of a trained professional. One of the best places to find a bariatric (weight-loss) physician is on the Web site for the American Society of Bariatric Physicians, www.asbp.org. Go to their home page and click "**For Patients.**" Under that heading click "**Find a Weight Loss Doctor.**" Then click your **state.** Your best choices will be under "**Certified by the American Board of Bariatric Medicine**" and/or "**American Society of Bariatric Physicians Bariatric Guidelines Compliant.**"

Let's Begin to Lose It Weight, That Is

Here are the steps for the weight-loss phase.

1. Use a meal-replacement shake or bar.
2. Eat a sensible meal.
3. Anti-inflammatory and antioxidant foods work.
4. Snack when hungry on healthy snacks.
5. Drink plenty of water.
6. Start an exercise program and get more active.
7. Get enough quality sleep.
8. Keep a journal or diary.
9. Be accountable and have a support system.

Use Meal Replacements

Meal replacements have been around for many years and come in the form of drinks, shakes, or bars. You simply replace one or two of your daily meals with these products.

The replacement meals offer the advantage of **portion control** and **stimuli narrowing**. In other words, they are a fixed amount of calories with minimal choices. There is no guesswork or trying to calculate how much you are eating, and over time this has been shown to be an excellent way of reducing calories and losing weight.[87]

A good meal replacement will have the following:

• fifteen to thirty grams of a complete protein per serving
• four to ten grams of fiber
• a low number of carbohydrates (a low glycemic load)
• three to five grams of a polyunsaturated fat (preferably an omega-3)
• 150 to 250 calories
• a good taste

Most are convenient to make or carry with you.

You can buy meal-replacement shakes commercially or make one yourself. To eight ounces of water, low-fat milk (fat-free or 1% milk), soy milk, almond milk, or coconut milk add a serving of protein powder. An excellent source of protein powder is whey isolate or whey concentrate, and that should be about fifteen to thirty grams of protein per serving. You may add fruit, like blueberries, or peanut butter. Blend and enjoy. These shakes can be quite good.

Most of the time people use meal replacements for breakfast and lunch. It is best not to use one during your family or social meal. Otherwise, you might feel deprived.

Eat a Sensible Meal

Lower-Fat Dieting

If you are using meal replacements for breakfast and lunch, then you need to have a sensible meal for supper. A sensible meal would be four hundred to five hundred calories with at least four to five ounces of protein (see Appendix B for a list of proteins). One ounce of cooked meat, chicken, or fish has about seven grams of protein, and you need about thirty grams per meal, which is four to five ounces.

In addition, your meal should include all the green vegetables you want. (We have never heard of anyone overdosing on broccoli.) Steamed or raw is best with some balsamic vinegar and olive oil for flavor and good fat.

Depending upon how much you need to lose and how strict your diet program is, you may add some fruit to your four-hundred-to-five-hundred-calorie meal. High-antioxidant fruits like blueberries, raspberries, etc., are a good choice (see Appendix C for a list of antioxidant foods).

By adding fruits and vegetables you are increasing your fiber consumption. Getting thirty to forty grams of fiber a day is essential for good health. Fiber is one of the best "colon cleanser" you can use, but a word of caution—start *slowly*. Work up to the higher amount of fiber over several weeks; otherwise, you will have gas, bloating, cramps, and some discomfort like a toxic plume hanging over you. You may need over-the-counter products like Beano or Gas-X to help with the problem.

In addition to foods, there are several commercially available fiber products (Metamucil™, Citrucel™, Benefiber™, to name a few). Make sure you use the ones sweetened with artificial sweeteners instead of sugar. Ask your pharmacist for some suggestions or purchase ground psyllium at a health-food store and add to food.

In the weight-loss phase, you should avoid or minimize yellow and orange fruits, which include bananas, oranges, pineapple, and cantaloupe. These are not bad fruits, but they have higher sugar contents and can be added back during maintenance. The best choices of fruits at this stage are berries—*blueberries*, which are high in antioxidants as well as being anti-inflammatory. In addition other forms of berries, cherries, apples, and pears are good choices.

Let's say a word about "white foods," which include white flour, sugar, rolls, bagels, donuts, potatoes, white rice, and anything else that is a "momma food" and tastes good. (*Just spit it out if it tastes good.*) You may *sparingly* eat these foods during maintenance as long as they don't cause weight gain. You want to *eliminate or severely restrict* them during the weight-loss phase, because they lack fiber and have a very high glycemic load, which makes them very inflammatory. These "white foods" raise your blood sugar too fast, thus causing a large spike of insulin, which sabotages your weight-loss efforts and perpetuates chronic inflammation and the "hostile takeover."

As mentioned previously, Barry Sears's "Anti-inflammatory Food Pyramid" can be found in Appendix D. The Zone Diet is an excellent anti-inflammatory way of eating. Simply put, it divides your plate into thirds. One-third should be your lean protein source and the other two-thirds should be vegetables. You can use olive oil on the vegetables for good fat. Fruit can be your dessert. Starches, breads, sugar, rice, potatoes, sweets, and other high-glycemic-load foods should be treated like condiments and used *very* sparingly, if at all. More about the "nuts and bolts" of a Zone Diet can be found in Dr. Sears' books *Toxic Fat, The Zone Diet*, and *The Anti-inflammatory Zone*.

Do you take your hands with you when you eat? If so, here is a "handy" chart to use when trying to figure out portion sizes.

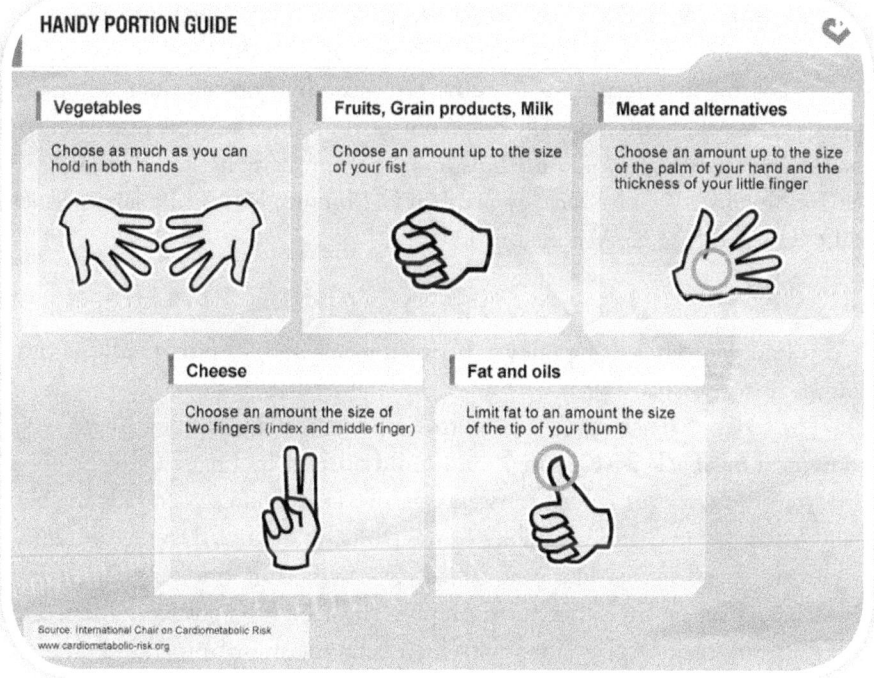

HANDY PORTION GUIDE

Vegetables
Choose as much as you can hold in both hands

Fruits, Grain products, Milk
Choose an amount up to the size of your fist

Meat and alternatives
Choose an amount up to the size of the palm of your hand and the thickness of your little finger

Cheese
Choose an amount the size of two fingers (index and middle finger)

Fat and oils
Limit fat to an amount the size of the tip of your thumb

Source: International Chair on Cardiometabolic Risk
www.cardiometabolic-risk.org

Lower-Carb Dieting

There is no question that a low-carbohydrate diet works best for rapid weight loss. Numerous studies have compared it to conventional diets, and hands down the low-carb diet works the fastest and is quite safe. The problem is that some people find it difficult to sustain this type of eating pattern. In addition, people don't know how to do a low-carb diet properly. **If you decide to be in the low-carb camp, you must stay in the low-carb camp. You cannot move from Mediterranean to low-carb back to Zone. It will not work.**

Contrary to popular belief, a low-carb diet is not a high-protein diet. You should eat about the same amount of protein as any other diet, and that should be about one hundred grams per day (four hundred kcal). You restrict carbohydrates to fifty grams per day (two hundred kcal) but no more than one hundred grams per day (four hundred kcal). Guess what? The rest of your daily calories *must* come from fat. In other words you are consuming 80 percent of your calories from fat. Fat will be in the form of butter, fat on meat, cream, olive oil, etc. If you have less than 60 percent of your calories from fat on these diets, they do not work well and there can be problems with your blood lipids and cholesterol.[88]

In addition, it takes two to three weeks for your body to adapt to a low-carb diet. Once you are adjusted, the diet works well and is safe. There are numerous studies proving its safety. Also, there are no restrictions on calories for low-carb diets, because they automatically help control your appetite (this is called ketosis, for you science geeks). For details on how to properly use the low-carb diet, see *The New Atkins for a New You,* by Stephen D. Phinney, MD, PhD; Jeff S. Volek, PhD, RD; and Eric C. Westman, MD.

Snack When Hungry

If you find yourself getting hungry between meals and/or hungry all the time, you may need to snack.

The types of snacks that help control appetite contain protein. **Always start your meal or snack with protein and build around it.** That should be about two to three ounces or fifteen to twenty grams. Lean-source protein is the best. In addition you may add vegetables or the fruits we discussed to the protein.

Avoid sugar snacks like candy, fruit by itself, fruit drinks, juices, sodas, chips, popcorn, or any other form of pure sugar or high-glycemic food. This will cause an insulin spike along with increasing inflammation and free-radical damage. Try these options:

- Peanut butter on vegetable sticks
- Greek yogurt (this is a higher protein choice)
- Fruit with cottage cheese
- Ten to fifteen unsalted raw or dry-roasted almonds or walnuts
- Lower-fat string cheese
- Meal-replacement shakes or bars with higher protein and lower carbohydrates.

One of our favorite snacks is ten to fifteen dry-roasted almonds along with one ounce of dark chocolate (70 percent cocoa). It makes you feel guilty, but it is so good.

Be aware of how hungry you really are. Follow this chart and only eat when you are a 4 or 5 on the hunger scale.

1. Stuffed	I do not want to eat again.
2. Satisfied/Full	I should have skipped the last few bites.
3. Comfortable/Neutral	I am not hungry or full.
4. Slightly Hungry	I suppose I could probably eat.
5. Very Hungry	Wow—I am hungry!
6. Famished/Dizzy/Faint	I am so hungry I could eat a horse!

Drink Plenty of Water

We recommend that you drink a half-ounce to one ounce of water daily for every pound you weight. If you weigh 120 pounds, you need between 60 and 120 ounces of water daily.

Water is necessary for hydration, better metabolism, weight control, bowel function, bladder function, temperature control, and good health. Bodily functions happen mostly in a water (aqueous) solution. Water is the universal solvent and vital for good health.

Let's take a moment and talk about another kind of drinking—alcohol. Remember, we said that alcohol is high in calories and must be first stored as fat before it can be released as energy. During the weight-loss phase of your program, you should avoid or severely restrict alcohol consumption. *Always drink responsibly.*

Many times when you think you are hungry, you are actually thirsty. Excess thirst can make you seem hungry and may cause you to overeat. So, if you are getting hungry during the day, try having a glass of water and see if that doesn't control your appetite. You might want to add a squeeze or two of lemon or lime to your water for antioxidants and flavor.

Also, athletes who are 1 to 2 percent dehydrated can lose up to 10 percent strength. Keep the fluids coming for maximal athletic performance.

Set me up for another round of water, please.

Start Exercising and Increase Your Activity

Nothing burns calories like muscle, and increasing muscle mass comes from exercising and adequate protein consumption.

See Chapter 6 on exercise and what exercise is right for you. **Also, before starting any exercise program, consult with your doctor.**

Start with twenty minutes a day if you are a beginner, and work your way to sixty minutes a day. Remember, you can divide the time into ten-to-fifteen-minute intervals throughout the day.

Remember NEAT activity is *unplanned* movement, and the more the better. You can do this by taking the stairs instead of the elevator, parking further away from the store, shop, or office, walking the long way around, taking the dog on a longer walk, and participating in daily activities rather than just watching.

So "move it or lose it." Maybe we should say, "Move it to lose it."

Get Enough Quality Sleep

Quality sleep is essential for good health and weight control, but sleep deprivation is clearly a problem in the United States:

> The average American sleeps 6.9 hours a night, which is less than the 7.5 to 8 hours of recommended sleep by experts. It is estimated that 30% to 40% of the U.S. population suffers occasionally from insomnia, and 10% to 15% have a chronic problem.
>
> ......
>
> Lack of sleep is directly linked to poor health, with new research suggesting it increases the risk of diabetes, heart disease, and obesity.[89]

In addition, a study published in the journal *Sleep* in 2004 found that women who averaged less than five hours of sleep had a higher death rate than those sleeping seven hours.

Even a few nights of bad sleep can be detrimental. One study found that people who were limited to three straight nights of sleeping five hours or less were more likely to have physical ailments such as headaches, stomach problems, and sore joints. Other studies have shown that curtailing sleep to four hours a night for several nights results in changes in metabolism that are similar to those that occur in normal aging and that raise levels of hormones linked with overeating and weight gain.

There is more "good" news.

Even when sleep deprivation does not cause illness or accidents, it can affect your quality of life. Sleep problems affect virtually every aspect of day-to-day living, such as your mood, mental alertness, work performance, and energy level. According to the 2005 NSF survey, almost three in ten working adults say they have missed work or made errors at work because of sleep-related issues in the past three months. And nearly one-fourth of partnered adults say they have sex less often or have lost interest in sex because they are too sleepy.[90]

As you can see, a good night's sleep is essential for good health and weight control. When you get less sleep, insulin resistance increases, and more of the cortisol hormone is produced from your adrenal glands. This hormone helps with stress and the fight-or-flight reaction you experience when being chased by a saber-toothed tiger. Since this usually does not happen in today's society, you just get all revved up with nowhere to go. Elevations of cortisol are designed for short-term use in your body, such as minutes or hours. When cortisol is chronically elevated over days, weeks, and months, chronic fatigue and overweight become a major problem.

So, the best advice is "go sleep it off."

Keep a Journal or Diary

Keeping a food journal helps prevent "food amnesia."

The problem with trying to remember what you ate is that the evidence disappears as you eat. *"What double hot fudge brownie?"* Keeping a journal or diary causes you to be accountable to yourself and to whoever will be reading it. Awareness is your key to success, and having a written paper trail helps keep you on track.

With that said, it is known in the weight-loss industry that food diaries are about 30 percent accurate, and people don't want to do them. Try keeping it for only two days during the week and one day during the weekend every month. Surely that is not too much, and by journaling intermittently, personal accountability and awareness can be yours.

Be Accountable and Have a Support System

If you have to show up somewhere and weigh in, your chances of being successful greatly increase. When you are going through the Stages of Behavioral Change[91] (see Chapter 2), time is necessary to make them permanent. Being accountable to someone is a great way of keeping you on track until you "own" that behavior.

Having a support system in place makes accountability easier. This can be in the form of a copilot (someone going through the same thing as you), a mentor, a teacher, a counselor, a church group, a weight-loss organization, a health-care professional, a personal trainer, or someone who has a vested financial interest in your success.

In addition, be a mentor to someone else. Take on a project to help another person struggling with the same problems you are. You would not want to disappoint them, so become a great supporting cheerleader for them. They in turn will do the same for you.

There is good news using modern day technology. A research study involving 348 people funded by the National Institute of Health found that those who logged into an interactive weight-loss maintenance Web site to record their weight at least once a month for 2.5 years maintained more weight loss than participants who logged in less frequently. One of the researchers stated, "If people use quality weight-management Web sites consistently, and they stick with their program, they are more likely to keep their weight off."[92]

Another study from the University of Texas Medical School published in 2010 found that:

> In conclusion, this Internet weight-loss community plays a prominent role in participants' weight-loss efforts—roles which might not be adequately filled by clinicians or offline family and friends. Internet-mediated support provides similar benefits as face-to-face support, with unique convenience, anonymity, and lack of judgment. Participants report that the support from this Internet community helps them lose weight as well as cope with being overweight. Social support within

Internet weight-loss communities merits further evaluation as a weight-loss resource for clinicians to recommend to patients.[93]

Here is something to think about. A great venue for accountability and support is a multi-level marketing (MLM) organization. With a simple program, a grassroots movement of accountability can form. Your sponsors have a vested interest in you being successful, and you want to be successful for the people you sponsor. With the right products and educational material, this may be an excellent way of combating the obesity epidemic.

10 Tips to Speed up Your Weight Loss

1. **Snack Smart.** Snacking for many people means mindlessly grazing throughout the day. Instead, prepare for midday hunger by having healthy snack options on hand. Look for low-fat options packed with protein, and try to find alternatives with a little bit of crunch. The most important thing is to plan ahead so that you never have to resort to eating the first thing you can get your hands on.

2. **Choose healthier condiments.** A lot of fat and sugar hides out in your condiments. Trade sugar for an artificial sweetener of your choice or agave nectar, and use mustard instead of mayonnaise. Order your low-fat salad dressing on the side, and dip your fork into the dressing instead of putting it on the salad; then you're more likely to use less. It's easy to forget about the calories and fat hidden in condiments because we only use a little at a time, but little changes that you're consistent with can lead to big losses at the scale.

3. **Walk. Walk. Walk.** Increasing exercise as you decrease your calories is proven to lead to weight loss. Take every opportunity to burn calories by walking. Take the stairs instead of the elevator, walk to the restaurant around the corner for lunch, and skip the parking spot right by the door.

4. **Anticipate temptation.** Be honest with yourself about what your weaknesses are, and plan ahead how you'll avoid them. If cakes and cookies are hard to resist, don't keep cake mixes or cookie boxes in your cupboard. If you're going to a holiday party, eat a healthy meal or snack beforehand to curb your appetite, or bring a diet buddy for support.

5. **Let your plate be your guide.** Use your plate to map out what you're eating. Fill two-thirds of your plate with vegetables and the other third with

protein (baked, boiled, or broiled) and **use a smaller plate or bowl.** If you refill your plate, stick with all vegetables.

6. Stay out of the drive-thru. Fast food is loaded with fat, sugars, and salt. You have very few healthy options on a fast-food menu, so your best bet is to avoid it all together. If you have to eat at a fast-food restaurant, refuse the super size and get baked or grilled instead of fried.

7. Be careful of what you drink. Stay away from sodas, sweet teas, and most fruit juices. You're better off eating an actual piece of fruit than sipping on the bottled juice cocktail made from concentrate. Opt for water or herbal teas whenever possible.

8. Be accountable. A lot of people will use a diet buddy or support group to keep themselves accountable for their diet and exercise choices. If you're choosing to go it alone, keep a detailed journal of what you eat and how much physical activity you're getting.

9. Eat out smart. Order smaller portions or share a plate with a friend to keep your portion sizes small when you go to a restaurant. Some people will put half of their meal in a doggy bag at the *beginning* of the meal, making sure they don't over eat the oversized portions served at most restaurants.

10. Acknowledge your success. Attitude is everything when it comes to the long journey of weight loss. Take time to recognize when you make healthy choices, and reinforce your positive behavior with rewards and affirmations.

Speeding up your weight loss is about putting together a lot of little changes to achieve big results.

Supplements

We need to say a few words about supplements. This includes vitamins, protein powders, meal replacements, nutraceuticals, etc.

First, when buying any over-the-counter (OTC) product, make sure that you get good quality with no contaminants. Only purchase products that have certified **GMP** stamped on the label. That stands for **Good Manufacturing Products.** GMPs are enforced in the United States by the Food and Drug Administration (FDA) and are a quality standard with which companies must comply. These standards are worldwide. If you don't see GMP stamped on a supplement, you probably should not buy it. One exception is pharmaceutical grade products. This labeling is a step above GMP and acceptable.

It has been said that if you eat the right foods you don't need vitamins and supplements. That is one big IF! Remember, we said that the ADA tells us that we should eat five to nine or more servings of fruits and vegetables a day, but the average American only eats 2.6 servings. This recommendation also supposes that the fruits and vegetables we are eating are of highest quality filled with all the good nutrients. *Good luck on that.*

Taking a certified GMP vitamin supplement is probably a good idea. As always, discuss this with your doctor.

Other supplements might be of benefit, too. For instance, calcium, vitamin D, omega-3 fish oils, curcumin, and coenzyme Q10 are examples. As always, before starting supplements, discuss them with your doctor, and make sure they are GMP certified.

You might be asking, instead of taking fish oil omega-3s, why not eat more fish. The answer is very simple. **Our fish are contaminated!** Dr. Barry Sears calls the fish supply "sewer of the sea."[94] There are too many PCPs, mercury, and other contaminants from industrial pollution. It is just a fact, as sad as that is. Appendix B gives you a list of the best choices of fish and seafood based on contamination.

Summary

We want to wish you success and happiness as you take your journey to having a healthier and leaner body. **Don't change the program, just stick with it.** Don't give up. You can be successful. You can be *radically free.*

Remember, everything starts with a healthy diet. You can take all the pills in the world, but unless your diet is correct, you are open to the attack of chronic inflammation led by the ringleader, NF-kB.

As you can see, these are very simple and basic steps like the little stars in the sky. Yet there is a tremendous amount of science backing up each one. By sticking to this program, go and find your "diamond in the sky."

"The proof of the pudding is in the tasting." This is an old saying that means "put up or shut up." Well, we are ready to "put up" and prove what we say works. Appendix E is a lifestyle-intervention study published by Dr. Kennedy and Dr. Warren in *The Bariatrician*, a medical weight-loss journal. Fifty people participated in a twelve-week weight-loss program. All fifty finished the program with an average weight loss of 31.3 pounds, a 5.8-inch reduction in waist circumference, and a 6.6 to 24.6 percent reduction in starting weight. These "Fab 50," as they were called, did a tremendous job. They are living proof that this system works. One year later 80 percent of the participants were still continuing on the program with an average weight loss of 44.5 pounds. **It works. Just follow the program like it is.**

It is now time for your commencement.

CHAPTER 9

Maintaining Your Weight

Welcome to your commencement.

The invitations have been sent, the crowds are gathering, and the ceremony is about to begin. Your cap and gown await you, but this commencement ceremony is different than most, because your life is the ceremony and your good health is your diploma.[95]

This is a new beginning in your life—a beginning of maintaining your weight loss. There is no end point or destination, because the journey is your destination. Never forget the difficulties of where you started. Celebrate life now as a healthier, happier person as you move on each day to higher levels of mastery in your journey. You are well trained; now use it.

The principles of maintenance are no different than the ones used to lose weight. They just have to be carried out for a longer time.

Defining Maintenance

A working definition of "maintenance" comes from the American Society of Bariatric Physicians and the National Institute of Health (NIH). Successful weight maintenance is defined as no more than a 6.6-pound (three kg) regain of your weight over two years following successful weight loss. Also, there must be a sustained reduction in waist circumference of at least 1.6 inches (four cm).

Once again, if you are a diabetic, maintenance must be at least four years, according to George Blackburn, MD, PhD, from Harvard Medical School.

Only by following good scientific principles and having accountability will you succeed. You want to prevent a lapse, relapse, and collapse. A lapse is a slight error or slip—the first instance of backsliding. A relapse occurs when lapses string together. A collapse occurs when relapse is complete and you return to "square one." You have been "seduced by the dark side."[96]

The "Dark Side" of Maintenance

"But beware of the dark side. . .If once you start down
the dark path, forever will it dominate your destiny."
—Yoda, *Star Wars*

We have all heard this kind of failure talk: "Each year an estimated 80 million Americans go on a diet, but no matter how much weight they lose, 95% gain it back within 5 years."[97]

Hearing this after or while dieting can be discouraging. You start to believe that the first three letters of the word "diet" tell you what people think of it. It is dying and deprivation. *"When you are on a diet you feel so righteous but deprived; off the diet you feel so guilty but relieved"*—and this seems to be people's perception.[98]

You start to feel like "It's too late for me, save yourself!"—the battle cry of too many dieters. Are you one of them? It doesn't have to be this way.

A minor slipup often propels us to misery. The guilt from a minor slip can make you susceptible to more slips and ultimately leads to loss of control and a collapse. This is definitely an example of "learned helplessness." You must not succumb to thinking, *"These things always happen to me; what's the use?"* Consider the lapse as an isolated incident, and that it will *not* interfere with your future successes.

"Past mistakes simply get you ready for future successes!"[99]

Here are six steps to mastering and preventing a lapse.[100]

1. **Stop, Look, and Listen:** A lapse is a signal of impending danger. Stop what you are doing and examine the situation. Look for alternatives, and listen to good advice like this book.
2. **Stay Calm:** If you get anxious or blame yourself, the situation can get worse. Take responsibility for your own actions, and be gentle and kind to yourself.
3. **Renew Your Vows:** Take a minute to remind yourself of how far you have come and how sad it would be if one silly little lapse canceled everything. Restate your goals and revisit the section on pain and pleasure in Chapter 2.
4. **Analyze the Lapse Situation:** Instead of blaming yourself, learn what things place you at risk for a lapse. Do certain feelings and environmental situations create risk? Eliminate them.
5. **Take Charge Immediately:** Leave the house or office if needed. Getting away from the situation may be the best alternative. Become proactive in making changes, and don't be reactive like in "learned helplessness."
6. **Ask for Help:** Call your coach or copilot for support, or see a professional. Do whatever it takes to prevent a lapse from becoming a relapse.

Be a "LOSER"

To understand how people have long-term success, we need to look at a bunch of "losers." The best place to find these losers is the National Weight Control Registry (NWCR), which was founded in 1993 and is a collaborative venture between James Hill, PhD, and Rena Wing, PhD.

To qualify for the NWCR, you must be at least eighteen years old and have successfully maintained a thirty-pound weight loss for a minimum of one year. To date there are over 10,000 members who have an average weight loss of seventy-one pounds and have maintained greater than a thirty-pound weight loss for 6.5 years.

About 80 percent of the participants from the NWCR are women with an average age of forty-five years who currently weigh on average 145 pounds.

Twenty percent are men with an average age of forty-nine years and average weight of 190 pounds.

At least 98 percent of the participants modify their diets in some way. The average calorie intake for women is 1,306 calories and for men is 1,685 calories. It should be noted that 78 percent of them eat breakfast.

In addition, 90 percent of the participants exercise for one hour every day, which burns about four hundred calories. Their most frequent exercises are:

Walking	76.6%
Weight lifting	20.3%
Cycling	20.6%
Aerobics	17.8%
Running	10.5%
Treadmill	6.3%
Stair climbing	9.3%

Their suggestions for sticking with exercise are to make it enjoyable and set realistic goals. Preplan where, when, and what you will do. Make sure you vary it. Also make it a regular routine in your life, and occasionally give yourself a break.

That is great advice from a "bunch of losers."

Myths about Long-Term Success[101]

Now let's explore some myths about long-term weight maintenance. If you plan to be a successful "loser" you need to dispel these myths.

Myth #1: Almost nobody who loses weight keeps it off.

This is not true. We know from the NWCR that people can be successful. Look at all those losers! The last data available showed 10,000 members maintained their weight for greater than 6.5 years. One study showed average weight losses of sixty-four pounds and average maintenance of eleven years. In fact, maintaining for two to five years decreases the risk of regain by over 50 percent.

Myth #2: If you were overweight as a child, it is impossible to lose weight and keep it off as an adult.

Approximately 46 percent of NWCR members were overweight by age eleven, 25 percent were overweight by ages twelve to eighteen, and 28 percent were overweight by age eighteen. Also, 46 percent of the members had one parent overweight, and 27 percent had both parents overweight.

Myth #3: To be successful at weight management, you have to be thin.

Many of the members are thinner, not thin. They are at a comfortable body weight, which is one at which they feel fairly good, given where they've been. They have no weight-related medical problems (metabolic syndrome, diabetes) and don't have to starve/exercise excessively to maintain.

Myth #4: There is no hope for yo-yo dieters.

Many of the participants of the registry have been on at least three to five diets. About 90 percent have lost weight many times before successfully maintaining their weight, bringing their total yo-yo weight loss to 270 pounds.

Myth #5: To lose weight and keep it off means a lifetime of suffering.

When the members were asked, "Do you feel like you are dieting?" nine out of ten said no. The overwhelming majority enjoy food, and seven out of ten eat in restaurants more than one or two times per week.

About three out of four members indicated that maintaining is easier or no harder than losing. The longer weight was kept off, the more likely it was to stay off.

When members were asked, "How do you handle cravings?" their answer was "Have a little." This is not about deprivation but about living a healthy lifestyle of balance and moderation.

This is a good place for a healthy chocolate snack to handle food cravings or mouth hunger, which is essentially the same thing.

Watch Out for Each Other's Well-Being

"Learning maintenance can be your greatest challenge. The trick is to prevent slips from occurring and to respond constructively when they do occur. Everyone makes mistakes, and the challenge is not to suffer CO-lapse."[102]

A lapse does not and must not lead to a relapse and collapse. Treat it for what it is—an unfortunate but *temporary* problem. Remember learned helplessness? You must not succumb to thinking, "*These things always happen to me; what's the use?*" Consider the incident or lapse as an isolated incident, and recovery will be quick.[103]

The guilt from a minor slip makes you susceptible to more slips and ultimately leads to loss of control and "being seduced by the dark side." It has been said that it takes a month to create a new habit and one to two years to make it permanent. During this time of formulating your new habit you are vulnerable to lapses. That is why a support system is vital for your maintenance.

Having a support group of several people who are going through the same maintenance issues is very beneficial. It helps to meet once a week or every other week for thirty minutes to an hour. You each stay accountable to each other, and mutual support strengthens each of you. Call each other between meetings to make sure you are on track. Also, if you are having a bad day, call for help. Being accountable to someone creates your strength. Become each other's wellness coaches.

You have probably heard the phrase "there is strength in numbers." Nothing could be truer in your journey to become forever fit. Getting a good support system is vital. You would not want to disappoint your partners, and they would not want to disappoint you. So, do it!

If there isn't a group available, find yourself a copilot—someone who is going through the same thing as you are. The two of you can make your own team. The important thing here is to have support.

Expectations

Having realistic expectations is crucial for long-term success.

Have you ever seen an advertisement that promises, "Lose thirty pounds in thirty days"? Do you think that is a reasonable expectation? Be honest. I know you wish it were true.

For some people who have massive amounts of weight to lose there is definitely hope for them besides surgery. In a study published in October 2010, it was reported that

> Among patients with severe obesity [Class II—BMI 35 or Class III— BMI 40, see Chapter I] a lifestyle intervention involving diet combined with initial or delayed initiation of physical activity resulted in clinically significant weight loss and favorable changes in cardio metabolic [heart disease] risk factors.[104]

There is definitely hope without surgery.

Accomplishing large amounts of weight loss might require being under the care of a bariatric physician. Remember that you can find one from the American Society of Bariatric Physicians Web site, at www.asbp.org, under find a physician in your state.

An interesting side note about severe obesity is that the most weight we have observed anyone lose in one week was thirty-seven pounds. That is not a typo. It is true, but the gentleman who lost this weight said it so well: "If you want to start at 475 pounds, you can lose that much in one week, too."

Have you or someone you know ever said, "I only lost one pound this week"? Only one pound! This seems to indicate that losing one pound is nothing. One pound of fat a week is a major accomplishment. You have to have a 3,500 calorie deficit (five hundred calories per day) for the week to lose that much. Cutting back five hundred calories a day is a big deal. That is a great job. Celebrate your successes and keep going. Don't fall into the trap of learned helplessness: *"Since I am not losing as fast as I want, I will just quit."*

Speaking of expectations, a classic study by Gary D. Foster, PhD, and Thomas A. Wadden, PhD, published in 1997 illustrates this all too well. It studied patients' views of what is a "reasonable" weight loss. Participants of the forty-eight-week weight loss trial were asked to define their "goal weight," "dream weight," "acceptable weight," and "disappointed weight."[105] The participants reported:

- Dream weight loss would be losing 32 percent.
- Happy weight loss would be losing 27 percent.
- Acceptable weight loss would be losing 25 percent.
- Disappointed weight loss would be losing 17 percent.

The actual weight loss of this group was 16 percent, which is tremendous, but it was below their "disappointed weight loss" expectations. In today's weight-loss arena, a 5 percent weight loss significantly reduces your risk for disease, and a 10 to 15 percent loss is "world class."[106]

The point is, get realistic expectations and celebrate your victories.

Commencement Speech from a Graduate

There is no better way to end this book than with a commencement speech from a graduate of the program. In fact, this is a very special graduate. His name is Guan Lim and he is a dear friend and business partner.

Guan has lost thirty-plus pounds. He simply said that he came to the realization that so many people he loved and cared about in his life were counting on him to be around (alive and healthy). He has seen too many people live undignified lives, making poor lifestyle choices, succumbing to a myriad of diseases due to being overweight, and dying way too young. Being overweight compromised his health and his ability to live a more active and productive life. So, he felt that shedding the unwanted weight and being healthy was the responsible and liberating thing to do, and he hopes to lead by example.

I am especially glad that he decided that he wanted to be around for his children, who are my adopted nieces and nephew, Jeremy, Nicole, and Michelle.

Guan remains successful to this day because of his determination and support groups of caring friends and family. His support group was and continues to be vital to his success, and your group can be vital to your success as well.

So take your diploma and continue your career of leanness. You owe it to yourself, your family, and your friends. No more excuses. Become *radically free* of the burden of overweight. It is time to get more out of life than obesity and disease. So, enough said. It's time to live. God bless!

To Be Continued...

APPENDIX A

Body Mass Index (BMI) Chart

BODY MASS INDEX

BMI (kg/m 2)	19	20	21	22	23	24	25	26	27	28	29	30	35	40
HEIGHT (IN.)				WEIGHT IN LBS										
58	91	96	100	105	110	115	119	124	129	134	138	143	167	191
59	94	99	104	109	114	119	124	128	133	138	143	148	173	198
5 ft 60	97	102	107	112	118	123	128	133	138	143	148	153	179	204
61	100	106	111	116	122	127	132	137	143	148	153	158	185	211
62	104	109	115	120	126	131	136	142	147	153	158	164	191	218
63	107	113	118	124	130	135	141	146	152	158	163	169	197	225
64	110	116	122	128	134	140	145	151	157	163	169	174	204	232
65	114	120	126	132	138	144	150	156	162	168	174	180	210	240
66	118	124	130	136	142	148	155	161	167	173	179	186	216	247
67	121	127	134	140	146	153	159	166	172	178	185	191	223	255
68	125	131	138	144	151	158	164	171	177	184	190	197	230	262
69	128	135	142	149	155	162	169	176	182	186	196	203	236	270
70	132	139	146	153	160	167	174	181	188	195	202	207	243	278
71	136	143	150	157	165	172	179	186	193	200	208	215	250	286
6 ft 72	140	147	154	162	169	177	184	191	199	206	213	221	258	294
73	144	151	159	166	174	182	189	197	204	212	219	227	265	302
74	148	155	163	171	179	186	194	202	210	218	225	233	272	311
75	152	160	168	176	184	192	200	208	216	224	232	240	279	319
76	156	164	172	180	189	197	205	213	221	230	238	246	287	328

RANGE	MEANING
less than 18.5	Underweight
18.5-24.9	Normal
25.0-29.9	Overweight
30.0-34.9	Obese
35.0-39.9	Severly Obese
40.0-50	Morbidly Obese
over 50	Super Obese

APPENDIX B

List of Proteins
(five-to-six-ounce portions)

Fish Based on Mercury Levels
The company Nordic Naturals[107] has compiled this list of mercury levels in fish.

Low Mercury (OK to Eat)

Arctic Cod	Anchovies	Butterfish
Catfish	Clam	Crab (domestic)
Crawfish/Crayfish	Flounder	Haddock (Atlantic)
Herring	Mackerel	Oyster
Salmon (canned, fresh, wild)	Sardine	Scallop
Shrimp	Sole	Squid
Tilapia	Trout	Whitefish

Radically Free

Medium Mercury (Eat Sparingly)

Bass (striped, black)	Carp	Cod (Alaskan)
Halibut (Pacific, Atlantic)	Lobster	Mahimahi
Monkfish	Perch/Sablefish/Snapper	Tuna (canned chunk light)
Sea Trout		

High Mercury (Avoid These Selections)

Bluefish	Crab (blue)	Grouper
Marlin	Orange roughy	Salmon (farmed, Atlantic)
Sea bass (Chilean)	Shark	Swordfish
Tilefish	Tuna (ahi, yellowfin, big eye, bluefin, canned albacore)	

Additional Sources of Protein

Cottage cheese (4–6 ounces) and low-fat cottage cheese	Nonfat cheese	Three large egg whites, or egg substitute
Sirloin (beef)	Beef—range fed	Buffalo—range fed
1.5 cups lentils, pinto beans, black beans, or other legumes	Chicken—white meat, no skin	Wild elk and wild deer

Vegetarian Choices

Soy burgers, soy hot dogs, soy sausage	Soybean Canadian bacon	Tofu

Monounsaturated Fat and Protein Foods

Almonds—whole, slivered, in butter or oil	Avocado	Cashews
Guacamole	Macadamia nuts	Olives and olive oil
Peanut butter, natural	Peanuts	

Meats should be baked, boiled, or broiled.
Protein portion size is five to six ounces.

APPENDIX C

List of Anti-inflammatory and High-Antioxidant Foods

Green Tea

Ginger

Garlic, onions, leeks, shallots, chives

Yams

Squash

Tomatoes

Persimmons

Beets (#I)

Mushrooms (shiitake, maitake, enokitake, cremini, Portobello, oyster, and thistle oyster)

Thyme

Turmeric and curry

Cruciform vegetables (cabbage, Brussels sprouts, bok choy, broccoli, cauliflower)

Carrots

Sweet potatoes

Pumpkins

Tomato sauce

Apricots

Soy

Rosemary

Oregano

103

Basil

Seaweed

Strawberries

Blueberries

Cranberries

Oranges

Lemons

Mint

Cinnamon

Raspberries

Blackberries

Dark chocolate (70 percent cocoa)

Tangerines

Grapefruit (be careful if taking some antibiotics and medications)

Pomegranate juice

APPENDIX D

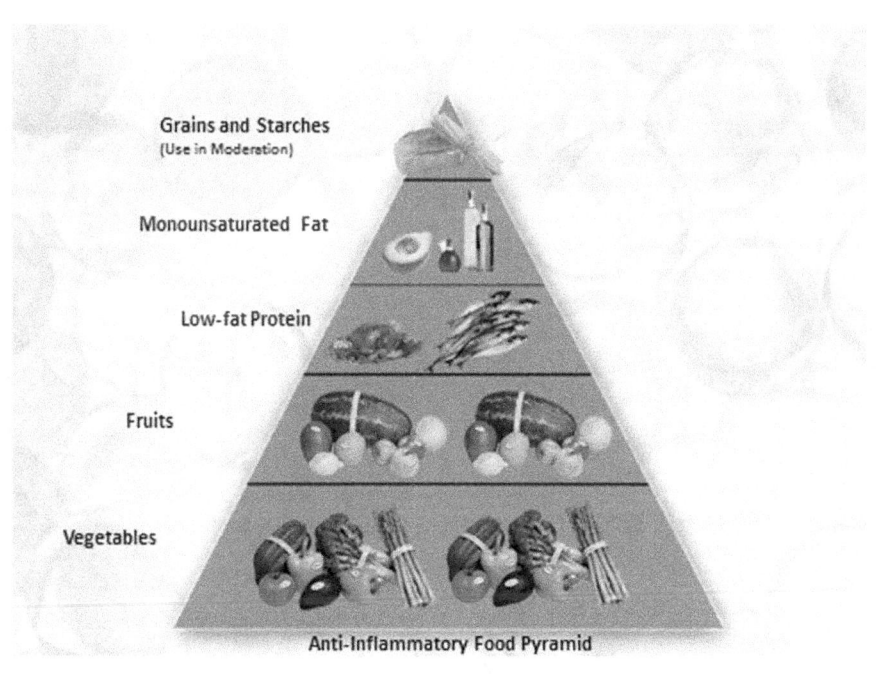

Anti-Inflammatory Food Pyramid

Courtesy of Barry Sears, PhD.

APPENDIX E

Weight-Loss Study Using a High-Antioxidant Cocoa Meal Replacement and Lifestyle Intervention

by
Machiel N. Kennedy, MD,
Diplomate ABFM and ABOM

Steven E. Warren, MD, DPA, CIME, FABFP, FABHPM, FAPWCA,
Diplomate ABFM

ABSTRACT

Context: Data supporting weight loss using a high-antioxidant meal replacement and lifestyle intervention are sparse.

Objective: To evaluate the effectiveness of a high-antioxidant meal replacement made from raw, unprocessed cocoa and lifestyle intervention over a twelve-week supervised weight-loss program.

Design, Setting and Participants: This was a lifestyle intervention trial. A high-antioxidant meal replacement was designed using raw, unprocessed cocoa with 8 grams of fiber, 21 grams of whey isolate protein, 3 grams of fat from chia oil, and 0.5 grams of sugar. The calories per meal replacement were 190 kcal, but the net calories were about 150 kcal. The participants ranged in age from twenty-six to seventy-three years. They were required to participate in a weekly support call with one of the physicians and consume two meal replacements a day and, for the third meal, eat a sensible, high-protein, low-carbohydrate meal of their choice totaling 1,200 kcal per day for women and 1,500 kcal per day for men. All of the fifty participants who started completed the study. Each was encouraged to exercise by at least walking. All participants had their meal replacements furnished, and monetary rewards were given to the winners of the group. The fifty participants were divided into groups of five, and the members of each group monitored each other in addition to the monitoring from the physicians and other staff on a weekly phone call.

Main Outcome Measures: Changes in weight, body mass index (BMI), and waist circumference were evaluated.

Results: Over a twelve-week period the average weight loss was 31.3 pounds with an average reduction in waist circumference of 5.8 inches. The percentage weight loss ranged from 6.6 percent to 24.6 percent of starting weight. There were no dropouts during the lifestyle intervention study.

Conclusion: Successful weight loss was achieved by using a high-antioxidant meal replacement made from raw, unprocessed cocoa along with a monitored program requiring accountability and lifestyle-intervention changes. In addition, furnishing product and rewarding participants for their behavior was successful in creating statistically significant weight loss in a group of overweight or obese subjects.

INTRODUCTION

The prevalence of obesity has risen markedly since 1976, now exceeding 30 percent among US adults. Obesity has well-known associations with morbidity and disability, resulting in unhealthy life-years and increased health-care costs. Currently in the US 68 percent of the population is either overweight or obese.[1]

The latest figures from the Centers for Disease Control (CDC) demonstrate that obesity continues to be a significant public health problem in the US. Note the list of health problems associated with weight.

- Coronary heart disease
- Type 2 diabetes
- Cancers (endometrial, breast, and colon)
- Hypertension (high blood pressure)
- Dyslipidemia (high total cholesterol or high levels of triglycerides)
- Stroke
- Liver and gallbladder disease
- Sleep apnea and respiratory problems
- Osteoarthritis
- Gynecological problems (abnormal menses, infertility, polycystic ovaries)

A very interesting quote from a 2010 article from M. D. Anderson Cancer Center talking about inflammation and cancer is:

> This indicates that lifestyle plays a major role in the development of cancer. The important lifestyle factors that affect the incidence and mortality of cancer include tobacco, alcohol, diet, obesity, infectious agents, environmental pollutants, and radiation. All of these risk factors are linked to each other through inflammation.[2]

---

[1] K. M. Flegal, M. D. Carrol, C. L Ogden, L. R. Curtin, "Prevalence and Trends in Obesity among US Adults, 1999–2008," *Journal of the American Medical Association* 303(3) (2010): 235–41.

[2] S. Sahdeo, et al, "Targeting Inflammatory Pathways by Flavonoids for Prevention and Treatment of Cancer," *Planta Medica* 76 (2010): 1044–63.

Since it is felt that obesity is related to oxidative stress and inflammation, a weight-control trial using a high-antioxidant meal replacement might be beneficial.

METHODS

Fifty people were chosen from over 250 applicants. Their age range was from twenty-six years to seventy-three years old. People on insulin therapy were excluded, and those with a major medical condition the physicians felt were inappropriate for the study were eliminated also.

The participants were either overweight or obese measured by BMI criteria set by the World Health Organization with >25 defining overweight and >30 defining obesity.[3]

Exclusionary criteria were insulin-dependent diabetes or any medical issue requiring medication that the physicians overseeing the study felt would not be appropriate.

The participants were to consume a high-antioxidant meal replacement shake made from raw, unprocessed cocoa by MXI Corporation. The shake had an ORAC FN score of 56,500 with 1,128 mg of flavonoids (certified by Brunswick Laboratories). One serving protected over five primary radicals, which was four times the USDA fruits/vegetables average.[4]

The shake was 190 kcal with 21 grams of whey isolate protein, 8 grams of fiber, 3 grams of fat from chia, and 0.5 grams of sugar. Each participant consumed two shakes a day for twelve weeks. In addition the participants consumed a 600-kcal meal. The total calories were 1,200 kcal per day for women and 1,500 kcal per day for men. Snacks consisted of chocolate squares or nuggets. If needed, participants could have a 200-kcal high-protein snack.[5]

The participants were encouraged to exercise by walking. They were to work their way up to ten thousand steps per day, and they could participate in

---

3 National Institute of Health, World Health Organization statistics on obesity.

4 Bell Advisory Services, David Bell, Brunswick Laboratories, New Bedford, MA.

5 G. L. Blackburn, "Making Scientific Sense of Different Dietary Approaches, Part-I: Evaluating the Diets. Part 2: Meeting Dietary Needs, Achieving Weight Loss," *Diabetes & Endocrinology* (2004) 6(1), accessed on *Medscape*.

more vigorous exercise if they desired and it was approved by their primary care physician.

Each participant was encouraged to get at least 7.5 hours of sleep per night.

Each participant was encouraged to get one ounce of water per pound body weight.

The fifty participants were divided into support groups of five people, and these groups participated in a physician call for thirty minutes once a week for the twelve weeks.

In addition, each participant completed a food and exercise journal and returned them by fax once a week. Included in the journal were their calorie consumption, amount of water consumed, a hunger chart, exercise completed, and amount of shakes taken.[6]

The meal-replacement shakes and a financial reward were given to the top "losers" of the group.

RESULTS

The average weight loss per participant was 31.3 pounds. In addition, there was an average decrease in waist circumference of 5.8 inches. None of the participants experienced any ill health from the program. The most common complaint was gastrointestinal upset and/or diarrhea.

COMMENTS

The combination of a high ORAC FN meal replacement made from raw, unprocessed cocoa along with a lifestyle-intervention program and financial rewards seems to be a highly effective way of achieving weight loss and weight control in overweight or obese individuals. Since both financial compensation and the lifestyle intervention were provided to all participants, the individual effects on weight loss of receiving monetary compensations versus the meal replacements cannot be determined.

_____

6   K. O. Hwang, et al, "Social Support in an Internet Weight-Loss Community," *International Journal of Medical Informatics* 79 (2010): 5–13.

While measurements of inflammatory markers associated with obesity and other diseases were not measured, it is hypothesized that they would have improved during the course of the study.

Previous testing using cell-based "efficacy" assays that were modified for testing natural products had shown that one serving of the meal replacement produced positive changes in inflammatory markers.[7] These tests use live cells to see whether or not products actually work to protect human cells. For the recent testing, anti-inflammation and antiaging tests, which use highly respected NF-kB and SIRT1 markers as performance standards, were selected, since both are believed to be involved in weight loss, glucose management, and a host of other wellness factors.[8] Both tests demonstrated positive results. A single serving of the meal replacement stimulates SIRT1 by approximately 15 percent and inhibits NF-kB by 34 percent. Furthermore, there are likely to be cumulative benefits that may result with regular daily consumption of the meal replacement.

ACKNOWLEDGEMENTS

The authors wish to thank MXI Corporation for supplying the meal-replacement shakes and financial rewards to the most successful participants.

REFERENCES

1) Flegal, K. M., M. D. Carrol, C. L. Ogden, and L. R. Curtin. ""Prevalence and Trends in Obesity among US Adults, 1999–2008." *Journal of the American Medical Association* 303(3) (2010): 235–41.

2) Sahdeo, S., et al. "Targeting Inflammatory Pathways by Flavonoids for Prevention and Treatment of Cancer." *Planta Medica* 76 (2010): 1044–63. M. D. Anderson Cancer Center, Houston, TX.

---

7   Bell Advisory Services, David Bell, Brunswick Laboratories. New Bedford, MA.

8   Sahdeo, et al, "Targeting Inflammatory Pathways," *Planta Medica* 76 (2010): 1044–63; C. G. Fraga, "Dark Chocolate May Improve Insulin Sensitivity/Resistance and Blood Pressure," *American Journal of Clinical Nutrition* 81 (2005): 541–2; N. Matsui, et al, "Ingested Cocoa Can Prevent High-Fat Diet-Induced Obesity by Regulating the Expression of Genes for Fatty Acid Metabolism," *Nutrition* 21 (2005): 594–601.

3) Blackburn, G. L. "Making Scientific Sense of Different Dietary Approaches. Part-I: Evaluating the Diets. Part 2: Meeting Dietary Needs, Achieving Weight Loss." *Diabetes & Endocrinology* (2004) 6(1). Accessed on *Medscape.*

4) Hwang, K. O., et al. "Social Support in an Internet Weight-Loss Community." *International Journal of Medical Informatics* 79 (2010): 5–13. Journal homepage: www.intl.elsevierhealth.com/journals/ijmi.

5) Fraga, C. G. "Dark Chocolate May Improve Insulin Sensitivity/ Resistance and Blood Pressure." *American Journal of Clinical Nutrition* 81 (2005): 541–2.

6) Matsui, N., et al. "Ingested Cocoa Can Prevent High-Fat Diet-Induced Obesity by Regulating the Expression of Genes for Fatty Acid Metabolism." *Nutrition* 21 (2005): 594–601.

BIOGRAPHY

Machiel Kennedy, MD, graduated from Indiana University Medical School and is board certified in family medicine and bariatric medicine. He has over thirty years' experience in clinical practice and weight-loss management. He has authored four books. The latest book was coauthored with Dr. Steve Warren and is titled *Radically Free: The Anti-inflammatory and Antioxidant Approach to Weight Management.* Dr. Kennedy was a consultant to MXI Corp for this study.

Steven Warren, MD, DPA, is a geriatric physician who is board certified in family medicine, hospice and palliative medicine, and wound care. He is in active practice in several long-term-care facilities. He has been doing research and lecturing on the health benefits of dark chocolate for the past six years. He owns a weight-loss clinic and is motivated to help people lose weight in order to help them avoid chronic health illnesses.

Reprinted by permission from the American Society of Bariatric Physicians (www.asbp.org) article as it appeared in the November 2011 edition of *The Bariatrician.*

INDEX

Cytokines 7, 48, 50, 54

D

Depression 13, 25, 26, 37, 58

Diabesity 8

Diabetes 1, 5, 7, 9, 10, 32, 33, 41,
 42, 47, 49, 51, 52, 53, 54, 57,
 58, 60, 82, 93, 109, 110

Diet 11, 30, 31, 32, 33, 35, 38, 42,
 45, 46, 47, 48, 49, 51, 52, 53,
 54, 57, 59, 60, 67, 78, 79, 80,
 85, 86, 87, 90, 92, 93, 95, 109,
 110, 112, 113

Dyer, Wayne 23

E

Eating Disorder (ED) 24, 25

Eicosanoids 47

Environment 42, 69, 70, 71, 73, 91, 109

Excuses 21, 22, 23, 67, 96

Exercise 11, 13, 15, 24, 25, 41, 53,
 63, 64, 65, 67, 77, 82, 85, 86,
 92, 93, 108, 110, 111

Expectations 27, 94, 95, 96

F

Fats 29, 30, 31, 33, 34, 35, 36, 37,
 44, 45, 49, 52, 54, 60

Fiber 30, 32, 77, 78, 79, 108, 110

Flavonoids 51, 56, 57, 109, 110, 112

Food and Drug Administration (FDA) 86

Franco, Oscar 46, 48

Free radicals 32, 48, 49, 50, 52, 53,
 54, 60, 61

Fruit 30, 36, 37, 38, 46, 51, 52, 53,
 55, 56, 59, 61, 77, 78, 79, 80,
 81, 86, 87, 110

Fuji Health Science 125

G

Gans, Keri 56

Generalized Anxiety Disorder 26

Ginger 58, 59, 60, 103

Glassman, Keri48

Glycemic index or load 32, 33, 44,
 52, 61, 77, 80

Goals 16, 17, 19, 21, 91, 92

Good Manufacturing Procedures
 (GMP) 86, 87

Gratifications 13, 14, 20

H

Habits 15, 19, 22, 24, 26

Healthy People 2010 2

Heart Disease 1, 4, 7, 9, 10, 32, 33,
 41, 45, 46, 47, 51, 52, 53, 54,
 57, 65, 82, 95, 109

Hostile takeover 6, 9, 43, 48, 49, 58,
 79

Hunger 81, 85, 93, 111

Hunger scale 81

I

Inflammation 9, 32, 41, 42, 43, 45,
 47, 49, 51, 53, 54, 55, 57, 59,
 61, 79, 80, 87, 109, 110, 112

Insulin Resistant Syndrome (IRS) 8,
 43, 48, 58, 83

J

Journaling 84

K

Kennedy, Machiel 87, 107, 113

REFERENCES

1   American Society of Bariatric Physicians Web site: http://www.ASBP.org.

2   National Health and Nutrition Examination Survey (NHANES) (2007–2008).

3   US Department of Health and Human Services, *Healthy People 2010* conference edition in 2 volumes (Washington, DC: US Department of Health and Human Services 2000). http://www.health.gov/healthypeople.

4   C. Wang, "Urgently needed: a framework convention for obesity control," *The Lancet*, vol. 378, issue 9793 (August 27, 2011).

5   Ibid.

6   National Cholesterol Education Program—Adult Treatment Panel III (NCEP-ATP III, 2005 guidelines).

7   E. S. Ford, W.H. Giles, and W.H. Dietz. "Prevalence of the Metabolic Syndrome among U.S. Adults: Findings from the Third National Health and Nutrition Examination Survey," *Journal of the American Medical Association* 287 (002): 356–359.

8   Martin E. P. Seligman, *Learned Optimism: How to Change Your Mind and Your Life* (New York: Free Press, 1990).

9   Martin E. P. Seligman, *Authentic Happiness* (New York: Free Press, 2002).

10   Ibid.

11   Ibid.

12   W. R. Miller and S. Rollnick, *Motivational Interviewing: Preparing People for Change* (New York: The Guilford Press, 2002).

13   Denis Waitley, *The Psychology of Winning: Ten Qualities of a Total Winner* (Chicago, IL: Berkeley Books, Nightingale-Conant, 1979).

14   Steven K. Scott, *A Millionaire's Notebook: How Ordinary People Can Achieve Extraordinary Success* (New York: A Fireside Book, 1996).

15   Miller and Rollnik, *Motivational Interviewing*.

16   Miller and Rollnik, *Motivational Interviewing*; Machiel Kennedy, *Ten Commitments to Be Forever Fit* (Bandon, OR: Robert D. Reed Publishers, 2005).

17   Miller and Rollnik, *Motivational Interviewing*.

18   "Convert dreams into goals, goals into tasks, and tasks into steps." Scott, *A Millionaire's Notebook*.

19   Seligman, *Learned Optimism*.

20   Ralph Carson, "Is Food an Addictive Substance?" (San Diego, CA: Presentation at the American Society of Bariatric Physicians Fifty-First Annual Obesity and Associated Conditions Symposium—Physicians Course, 2001).

21   Tom Massey, *The ABC's of Successful Living: Getting What You Really Want* (San Francisco, CA: Robert D. Reed Publishers, 2001).

22   Carson, "Is Food an Addictive Substance?"

23   Massey, *The ABC's of Successful Living*.

24   Unless otherwise noted, the defined disorders below are taken from Max Hamilton's *Comprehensive Textbook of Psychiatry*, 1B, volume 1, fifth edition (Kaplan & Sadock); and *DSM-IV-TR Diagnostic and Statistical Manual of Mental Disorders* (American Psychiatric Association).

25   Wikipedia, s.v. "Eating Disorders," last modified April 16, 2012, http://en.wikipedia.org/wiki/Eating_Disorders.

26   Hamilton, *Comprehensive Textbook of Psychiatry*.

27   Paul T. Mason and Randi Kreger, *Stop Walking on Eggshells: Taking Your Life Back When Someone You Care about Has Borderline Personality Disorder* (Oakland, CA: New Harbinger Publications, Inc., 1998).

28   J. H. O'Keefe, et al, "Dietary Strategies for Improving Post-Prandial Glucose, Lipids, Inflammation, and Cardiovascular Health," *Journal of the American College of Cardiology* 51(3) (2008). Accessed on *Medscape* medical news.

29   American Society of Bariatric Physicians speaker on protein.

30   "Silent inflammation" is a term attributed to Dr. Barry Sears, author of *The Zone Diet*.

31   S. Sahdeo, et al, "Targeting Inflammatory Pathways by Flavonoids for Prevention and Treatment of Cancer," *Planta Medica* 76 (2010): 1044–63.

32   Barry Sears, *Toxic Fat: When Good Fat Turns Bad* (Nashville, TN: Thomas Nelson, Inc., 2008).

References

33   Ibid.

34   David Servan-Schreiber, *Anticancer: A New Way of Life* (New York: Penguin Group, 2008).

35   Ibid.

36   D. Mann, "Days of Wine and Chocolate (and Fish, Almonds, and Garlic) Might Cut Heart Risk by More Than 75%," *Medscape* (December 18, 2004). http://www.medscape.com/viewarticle/538065

37   Ibid.

38   Keri Glassman, *The O₂ Diet: The Cutting-Edge Antioxidant-Based Program That Will Make You Healthy, Thin, and Beautiful* (New York: Rodale Books, 2010).

39   Barry Sears, *The Anti-Inflammation Zone: Reversing the Silent Epidemic That's Destroying Our Health* (New York: Regan Books, 2005).

40   Sears, *Toxic Fat.*

41   George Lucas, *Star Wars.*

42   Sahdeo, et al, "Targeting Inflammatory Pathways," *Planta Medica* 76 (2010): 1044–1063.

43   C. Weatherby, "Good-bye Vioxx, Hello Anti-Inflammatory Foods: "Silent" Inflammation Drives Aging, and Drugs Aren't the Only—or Best—Remedies," *Vital Choice Seafood Newsletter* (November 12, 2004) Article 0000326609.

44   *Wikipedia*, s.v. "Antioxidant," last modified April 10, 2012, http://en.wikipedia.org/wiki/Antioxidant.

45   Hershey's, "Antioxidants," http://www.thehersheycompany.com/nutrition-and-wellness/chocolate-101/antioxidants.aspx.

46   Sahdeo, et al, "Targeting Inflammatory Pathways," *Planta Medica* 76 (2010): 1044–1063.

47   O'Keefe, et al, "Dietary Strategies." http://www.medscape.com/viewarticle/569077.

48   Ibid.

49   H. K. Choi, "Fructose-Rich Beverages and Risk of Gout in Women," *Journal of the American Medical Association*, Vol. 304, No. 20 (November 24, 2010): 2270–78.

50   M. Shargorodsky, et al, "Effect of Long-term Treatment with Antioxidants (Vitamin C, Vitamin E, Coenzyme Q10 and Selenium) on Arterial Compliance: Humoral Factors and Inflammatory Markers in Patients with Multiple Cardiovascular Risk Factors," *Nutrition and Metabolism* 7(55) (2010).

51 National Health and Nutrition Examination Survey (NHANES) (2007–2008).

52 Sears, *The Anti-Inflammation Zone*; Wikipedia.

53 R. Prior, J. Joseph, G. Cao, B. Skukitt-Hale, and J. Mayer, Human Nutrition Research Center on Aging at Tufts, Boston, Agricultural Research Service, United States Department of Agriculture (1999). http://ars.usda.gov/is/pr/1999/990208.htm?pf=1.

54 Wikipedia, s.v. "Oxygen Radical Absorbance Capacity," last modified April 7, 2012, http://en.wikipedia.org/wiki/Oxygen_radical_absorbance_capacity.

55 C. G. Fraga, "Dark Chocolate May Improve Insulin Sensitivity/Resistance and Blood Pressure," *American Journal of Clinical Nutrition* 81 (2005): 541–2, 611–14. Accessed on *Medscape* medical news. http://www.medscape.com/viewarticle/501333.

56 Cal Orey, *The Healing Powers of Chocolate* (New York: Kensington Publishing Corp., 2010).

57 Wikipedia, s.v. "Health Effects of Chocolate," last modified February 8, 2012. http://en.wikipedia.org/wiki/Health_effects_of_chocolate.

58 Kennedy, *Ten Commitments to Be Forever Fit.*

59 G. Nemecz, "The Health Benefits of Dark Chocolate," *U.S. Pharmacist* Vol. 29:02 (posted 2/15/2004). http://www.uspharmicist.com/oldformat.asp?url=publish/content/8_1210.htm.

60 A. J. Flammer, et al, "Dark Chocolate Improves Coronary Vasomotion and Reduces Platelet Reactivity," *Circulation* 116 (2007): 2376–82.

61 N. Matsui, et al, "Ingested Cocoa Can Prevent High-Fat Diet-Induced Obesity by Regulating the Expression of Genes for Fatty Acid Metabolism," *Nutrition* 21 (2005): 594–601.

62 L. Iversen, *The Science of Marijuana* (New York: Oxford University Press, Inc., 2008); L. Barclay, "Dark Chocolate May Improve Insulin Sensitivity/Resistance and Blood Pressure," *American Journal of Clinical Nutrition* 81 (2005): 541–2, 611–14; A. J. Flammer, et al, "Dark Chocolate Improves Coronary Vasomotion," *Circulation* 116 (2007): 2376–82; N. K. Hollenberg and N. D. L. Fisher, "Is It the Dark in Dark Chocolate?" *Circulation* 116 (2007): 2360-62; N. Rose, "Mood Food: Chocolate and Depressive Symptoms in a Cross-sectional Analysis," *Archives of Internal Medicine* 170(8) (2010): 699–703.

References

63   E. T. Massolt, et al, "Appetite Suppression through Smelling Dark Chocolate Correlates with Changes in Ghrelin in Young Women. *Regulatory Peptides* (2010), doi: 10.1016/j.regpep.2010.01.005.

64   Bharat Aggarwal, "Targeting Inflammation-Induced Obesity and Metabolic Diseases by Curcumin and Other Nutraceuticals," *Annual Review of Nutrition* 30 (2010): 14.1–14.27, doi: 10.1146/annurev.nutr012809.104755.

65   Ibid.

66   K. Hughes, *The Incense Bible* (New York: Haworth Press, 2007).

67   According to the National Cancer Institute.

68   K. Yazawa, *Astaxanthin for Beautiful Skin, Eye Health, and a Sharp Brain* (Heart Publishing Co., LTD., 2007).

69   Ibid.

70   Fuji Health Science, "About Astaxanthin." http://www.fujihealthscience.com/astaxanthin.html.

71   American College of Sports Medicine, *ACSM's Guidelines for Exercise Testing and Prescription*, eighth edition (Baltimore, MD: Lippincott Williams & Wilkins, 2010).

72   J. A. Levine, S. J. Schleusnerr, and M. D. Jensen, "Energy Expenditure of Non-exercise Activity," *American Journal of Clinical Nutrition* 72 (2000): 1451.

73   *ACSM's Guidelines for Exercise Testing and Prescription.*

74   Ibid.

75   Ibid.

76   T. S. Church, et al, "Effects of Aerobic and Resistance Training on Hemoglobin A_{1C} Levels in Patients With Type 2 Diabetes," *Journal of the American Medical Association*, Vol. 304, No. 20. (November 24, 2010): 2253–62.

77   Kelly D. Brownell and Thomas A. Wadden, *The LEARN Program for Weight Control* (Dallas, TX: American Health Publishing Company, 1998).

78   Brian Wansink, "Food for Thought: An Inside Look at Food Psychology and the Unconscious Factors Causing People to Overeat," (Omaha, NE; Wellness Councils of America expert interview, 2004), http://www.welcoa.org/freeresources/index.php?category=16.

79   Kennedy, *Ten Commitments to Be Forever Fit.*

80   Allan Borushek, *The Doctor's Pocket Calorie Fat & Carbohydrate Counter* (Costa Mesa, CA: Family Health Publications, 2004), www.calorieking.com; Kennedy, *Ten Commitments to Be Forever Fit.*

81 Wansink, "Food for Thought," http://www.welcoa.org/freeresources/index.php?category=16.

82 Ibid.

83 Eric Schlosser, *Fast Food Nation: The Dark Side of the All-American Meal* (New York: Perennial, an Imprint of Harper Collins Publishers, 2002).

84 Ibid.

85 Wansink, Food for Thought," http://www.welcoa.org/freeresources/index.php?category=16.

86 These are the recommendations of the American Society of Bariatric Physicians (http://www.ASBP.org) and of G. L. Blackburn's article "Making Scientific Sense of Different Dietary Approaches. Part-1: Evaluating the Diets. Part 2: Meeting Dietary Needs, Achieving Weight Loss," *Diabetes & Endocrinology* 6(1) (2004), accessed on *Medscape.*

87 G. L. Blackburn, "Making Scientific Sense of Different Dietary Approaches," *Diabetes & Endocrinology* 6(1) (2004), accessed on *Medscape.*

88 J. S. Volek and S. D. Phinney, *The Art and Science of Low Carbohydrate Living* (Beyond Obesity, LLC, 2011).

89 Lawrence J. Epstein and Steven Mardon, *The Harvard Medical School Guide to a Good Night's Sleep* (New York: McGraw-Hill Companies, 2007).

90 Ibid.

91 The Stages of Behavioral Change are pre-contemplation, contemplation, preparation, action, maintenance, and termination. See p. 24–25.

92 *Journal of Medical Internet Research* study published in advance of August 2010. Funded by a grant from National Institute of Health.

93 K. O. Hwang, et al, "Social Support in an Internet Weight-Loss Community," *International Journal of Medical Informatics* 79 (2010): 5–13.

94 Sears, *Toxic Fat.*

95 Kennedy, *Ten Commitments to Be Forever Fit.*

96 Lucas, *Star Wars.*

97 *Time* magazine, 1/16/95.

98 Kennedy, *Ten Commitments to Be Forever Fit.*

99 Ibid.

100 These are taken from the American Board of Bariatric Medicine 1999 and 2000 Review Course and from Machiel Kennedy's book *Ten Commitments to Be Forever Fit.*

101 The myths are taken from *ACSM's Guidelines for Exercise Testing and Prescription* (Baltimore, MD: Lippincott Williams & Wilkins, 2010).

References

102 Kennedy, *Ten Commitments to Be Forever Fit.*

103 Seligman, *Learned Optimism;* Kennedy, *Ten Commitments to Be Forever Fit.*

104 B. H. Goodpaster, et al, "Effects of Diet and Physical Activity Interventions on Weight Loss and Cardiometabolic Risk Factors in Severely Obese Adults," *Journal of the American Medical Association,* Vol. 304, No. 16, (October 27, 2010): 1795–1802.

105 G. D. Foster, T. A. Wadden, R. A. Vogt, G. Brewer, "What Is a Reasonable Weight Loss? Patients' Expectations and Evaluations of Obesity Treatment Outcomes," *Journal of Consulting and Clinical Psychology,* Vol. 65 (1) (February 1997): 79–85.

106 According to the American Society of Bariatric Physicians Web site (www. ASBP.org), the Obesity Society Web site (www.obesity.org), and G. D. Foster, et al, "What Is a Reasonable Weight Loss?" *Journal of Consulting and Clinical Psychology,* Vol. 65 (1) (February 1997): 79–85.

107 http://www.nordicnaturals.com or http://www.nrdc.org.

www.ingramcontent.com/pod-product-compliance
Lightning Source LLC
Chambersburg PA
CBHW070146290526
45789CB00002B/648